GET BACK UP

HOW TO SOLVE BACK PAIN AND RECLAIM YOUR LIFE

By Dr. Erik Gullen, PT, DPT & Dr. Matt Klingler, PT, DPT

Copyright © 2021 by Dr. Erik Gullen PT, DPT & Dr. Matt Klingler PT, DPT
All rights reserved.
ISBN: 9798591046576

Village Fitness And Physical Therapy, INC.
146 North Glendora Avenue Suite 106, Glendora, CA 91741

(626) 385-8844

getbackupbook.net
villagefpt.com

Table of Contents

Acknowledgments	7
Before You Get Started	8
Introduction: The New Normal	8
Part 1: Why You Have Back Pain	**13**
Chapter 1: Modern Medicine's Failure to Address Low Back Pain	15
For All Its Naughtiness, Sometimes Modern Medicine Is Nice...	20
Chapter 2: The Inflammastories	21
Bodville, USA	21
The Allegory	23
Boddington Castle	26
Life Is A Highway	27
Sacred Ice Cream	28
Cup O' Inflammation	29
Life and Pain	29
The Nonlinear Path	30
Skill vs. Material	30
Butch Cartilage and the Trust Fund Kid	31
Chapter 3: Turning Pain Science Into Plain Science	33
The Sensation-Threat-Danger-Alarm-Pain-Action System	35
What If You Didn't Feel Pain?	36
Chapter 4: Structural Integrity	43
What Are Discs?	43
What Are Bones and Joints?	45
What Are Nerves?	46
What Are Muscles?	46
What Is Skin?	47
Chapter 5: Dubious Diagnoses	49
What Is Sciatica?	50
What Is a Muscle Spasm?	51
What Is a Disc Bulge, Rupture, Herniation, Slip, or Protrusion?	51
Scoliosis/Leg Length Discrepancies	52
What Is a Lumbar Strain?	53
What Is Chronic Injury?	54
What Is Chronic Pain?	55
What Is Fibromyalgia?	56
What Is Degenerative Disc Disease?	57
What Is Spondylolisthesis?	57
MRIs, X-Rays, CT Scans, and Other Imaging	58
Is This a Medical Emergency?	59
When It's Time to Get In to See Your Doc ASAP	60

Part 2: The Plan — 61

Chapter 6: Prognosis — 63
- "How long will this take to get better?" — 63
- Do You Believe That You Can Get Better? — 64
- Finding Your Flight Plan — 65
- The Healing Human Body — 66
- What to Do to Help Your Body Heal Faster — 66

Chapter 7: The Get Back Up Foundations Program — 69
- A Preface to the Foundations Program — 69
- Get Back Up Foundations Program — 70
- Exercises — 84
  - Supine — 84
  - Prone — 89
  - Sidelying — 93
  - Quadruped — 98
  - Sitting — 103
  - Standing — 110
- What If I Complete Phase 1 and Still Have Pain? — 116
- What's Next? — 116

Chapter 8: Balls, Core, And Stretches Galore — 117
- Using Mobility Tools To Beat Back Pain — 118
- Stretches For Beating Back Pain — 131
- Band Stretches — 142
- Back Pain Core Routine — 147

Part 3: The Principles — 153

Chapter 9: The Village Principles — 155
Chapter 10: Control Carbs — 157
Chapter 11: Eat Healthy Fats — 159
Chapter 12: Prioritize Veggies — 161
Chapter 13: Source Responsibly — 165
Chapter 14: Rest Deeply — 169
Chapter 15: Get Outside — 171
Chapter 16: Solve Pain — 173
Chapter 17: Don't Go It Alone — 177
Chapter 18: Build Strength For Longevity — 179
Chapter 19: Escape The Sedentary — 183
Chapter 20: Breathe Freely — 185
Chapter 21: Attain Alignment — 189
Chapter 22: It's OK To Ask For Help — 193
- Why Is a Coach Essential for Getting Out of Pain? — 193
- Do You Want Our Help? — 193

Conclusion	**195**
Appendix: Frequently Asked Questions	**197**
Who Can Help Me?	197
Should I Get a Massage?	198
Should I Do Chiro?	198
Should I See a PT?	199
Should I Go to My Primary Care?	199
How Can I Exercise If Everything Hurts?	200
Should I Do Mobility Exercises Like Foam Rolling and Stretching?	200
Should I Do High-Intensity Exercise?	201
Should I Do Cardio?	202
How Will Breathing/Breathing Exercises Change Back Pain?	203
How Can I Make My Core Really Strong?	204
How Can I Fix Alignment in My Body? How Does Neutrality Affect Back Pain? How Can I Get My Body Neutral?	204
About The Authors	**205**
Health Advice Disclaimer	**207**

Acknowledgments

Thanks to D.M. for letting us use your cabin as a writing retreat to power through and finish this book. Thanks to our amazing staff and clients who inspire us to continue to grow, develop, and create resources like this one. Carmen Singleton, thanks for taking stellar photos. Marky, Mark Miller (please don't edit how I spelled your name), you are an encouraging editor. Thanks to Ethan Bailey for letting us look over his shoulder and criticize his every design move. And thanks to Nicole and Krissy, our lovely wives, for their love and support.

Before You Get Started

Go to getbackupbook.net and download the FREE resources associated with this book. You'll find videos of EVERY exercise in the plan section and a bunch of awesome resources.

Introduction: The New Normal

It's everywhere and everyone's doing it. We see back pain in our families, in our workplaces, in our golfing buddies. It's not just everyday Joe and Jane who have back pain. It's also Joe's doctor, and his doctor's assistant, even the nurses at the clinic he goes to. Its ubiquitousness makes it feel normal, an inevitable part of life, perhaps even a rite of passage. We laugh it off as part of getting old. We follow a well worn path to address it: First, it's over-the-counter pain pills and generally "taking it easy." Next, it's choosing certain types of chairs, buying inversion tables, and maybe even shelling out a few thousand dollars to install a jacuzzi in the backyard. Eventually, so much of our behavior has changed that our understanding of who we are begins to change. Someone who thinks of themselves as active and healthy may begin to look in the mirror and accept a fearful, more sedentary version of themselves.

Back pain is a bully who plays a long, vicious game against not only our bodies but also our minds and spirits. At the end of this bleak road is surgery. It would not be our first choice. It would not be our 100th choice. But after the back pain bully has worn down our bodies and spirits, we are open to the idea of surgery. Risky? Check. Expensive? Check. Effective? Just like Congress. "But I guess it's the only option... Well, there were those people who wave healing crystals in Santa Monica... and I have been wanting a nice beach day... I could bring an umbrella and some snacks... I wonder if there is any takeout left in the fridge... Thought trains are weird... What was I thinking about? Oh yeah... back surgery. Yikes. I'm going to go drown my sorrows in leftover takeout..."

Why are some injuries mere inconveniences while others are living nightmares? Think of the last time you sprained your ankle. It was painful. It was swollen. It made it difficult or impossible to walk and exercise for a few weeks. But chances are it never scared you. Eventually it healed and you got on with life.

Compare that to your low back pain. Yeah, maybe it hurts and makes it hard to move. But there is another level to it, a sort of paranoia: "Do I have a herniated disc? I remember when my uncle did that and he had to get surgery... I saw my MRI and they said I have terrible arthritis. Am I going to end up like my dad and be in a wheelchair? Will I have to slow down and miss out on life and the joy of retirement? I've heard of people who threw out their back and then couldn't feel their feet anymore... Will this last forever? Should I see a chiropractor? An acupuncturist? My doctor? Physical therapist? Massage?" You might even start to beat yourself up: "I should have stretched more! I've really let myself go! This proves I'm getting old!"

Suddenly, what should be a simple, treatable problem becomes a monster, and it's all because of one thing: The Unknown.

When you sprain an ankle or even fracture a bone in the arm or leg, you can see exactly what happened. There is no mystery. There are no big questions. There is no unknown. There is just a smarting wound, a brace or cast, and a couple weeks of waiting.

Back pain is a phenomenon not unlike the little boy terrified of the boogeyman in the closet. As soon as mom or dad opens the door, peers inside, and confirms, "No boogeyman here!" the child's fear subsides and he falls asleep. Unfortunately, most folks going to the doctor's office leave with images of oozing jelly donut discs in their heads and prescriptions for narcotic pills in their pockets. Rather than a sense of encouragement and confidence in the healing journey, folks are filled with worry. It's the fear, not the original injury, that sets so many people up for chronic, debilitating pain. It is a terrible irony.

But it can be different for you. We wrote this book to give you the facts and relieve your fears.

We want your story to be far different from the sad reality that most people with back pain face (an endless stream of pills, injections, surgeries, and the loss of independence and mobility). We want your story instead to be one of beating back pain and living a healthy, active life like the thousands of clients we've helped.

We want you to be like Ron. Ron is in his late 50s and has worked his way up in a steel company over the last 30 years. Now he manages a team of people and a lot of stress. He has worked hard to provide for his family and put his two kids through college. With enough money to retire in the next few years, Ron was looking forward to enjoying the payoff from all his years of toil. But his low back pain was threatening to ruin the dream. Every time Ron would stand up, he would limp for the first few minutes because of the sharp pain in his back. The pain was so bad that he was on the brink of surgery when he started working with us. We were his "last hope." Using the exact principles laid out in this book, Ron was able not only to get out of back pain but also to get active again, lose 30 pounds, and rediscover his passion for surfing!

Unlike Ron, Charlene, who was 62, came to us after she'd already had low back surgery. Sadly, it didn't make her pain go away, and she was left taking a litany of medications, which left her with side effects like weight gain, lightheadedness, and made it difficult to focus. Charlene's daughter had recently said a simple sentence that motivated her to take action: "Mom, I don't want to eat at that restaurant because they don't have close parking, and I don't want you to have to walk that far." Charlene was mortified at the thought of her family having to change plans because of her limitations. She didn't want to slow down. She didn't want to lose her independence and mobility. She didn't want to give up. So Charlene came to us ready for change. Within a few months, using the exact principles laid out in this book, she was losing weight, noticed her back pain improving, and was starting to exercise again. Fast forward a year later, and she's in the best shape she's been in for the last 30 years, has lost

50 pounds, and feels amazing.

This book is for commuters and C-level execs like Frank. When Frank first came to us, he had pulled his back while doing rows at the gym. It was so bad that he had to cancel a big work trip. For Frank, cancelling work meant missing out on potential revenue for the business, and he was willing to do anything to get his back working again. After working with our team here at Village, he was not only back to working and working out, but he learned WHY his back pain started and WHAT to do so it was less likely to come back in the future. Heck, he even lost a few pounds in the process by implementing the nutrition habits we lay out in Part 3.

This book is for teachers with chronic pain like Sam. Sam had been bounced around to various health professionals, looking for a solution to her low back pain for nearly a decade. Her pain was so bad that she was having difficulty sitting for more than a few minutes at a time. It's nearly impossible to grade papers when you can't even sit. But after a few months here at Village, she was fully engaged in a workout routine, sitting with ease, and amazed at her progress. Using the exact principles we lay out in this book, Sam was able to decrease the FEAR associated with her low back pain and get her life back.

This book is for Dan, a paramedic in his 50s who was fearful he would need to retire early because of his low back pain. His pain came on while lifting patients and when he was in awkward positions at work. Since lifting and being in awkward positions are an unavoidable part of being a paramedic, he had to push through. For Dan, the solution to his back pain was much simpler than he thought it would be. Within a few months of being at Village, he was working pain free and ecstatic about his progress.

Why aren't there more success stories like these? Well, as we will talk about in Chapter 1, the medical world today is set up in a way that makes getting out of back pain nearly impossible. But even before getting caught up in the dysfunctional medical industry, people are often caught up in their own personal body dissonance.

Most body-owners choose to deny their own significance. Some become wildly self-centered, choosing to indulge every impulse until their bodies are polluted and destroyed by excess. These people are often young. Others become self-centered in more subtle ways: They may refuse a hundred tiny disciplines over and over until one day they become dependent on others, including their own children, nursing homes, or government programs. These people are often older. Still others don't seem to be very selfish at all. Quite the opposite. They are the ones who seem to deny themselves at every turn, saying yes to every call to service, volunteer opportunity, and cry for help. These folks are in every age and stage of life.

It is the mother who invests every ounce of time and energy into her kids, not realizing that the greatest thing she can give her precious children is an example of a healthy adult person.

It is the wealthy businessperson who donates considerably to charity or the beloved local minister, who both work so much that they rarely see their own families.

It is the retiree who saves and saves and saves for a big vacation with their spouse, but has to cancel at the last minute because their sciatic pain was so bad.

Learning how to fix your back pain not only involves cutting-edge healing arts but also a firm belief in the value of your own life. As you read through the specifics in this book, make it your mantra also to cultivate a strong, durable, growing love for life — the kind that is impossible not to share with those around you. For that is what life does: It grows. It shares. It gives. If you do that, all the information in this book will become exponentially more useful.

Part 1: Why You Have Back Pain

Chapter 1: Modern Medicine's Failure to Address Low Back Pain

If you are reading this book, you or someone you know (or maybe both of you) have back pain. It may not surprise you to learn that low back pain is one of the top ten causes of disability in the entire world. In fact, it is numero uno in Years Lived with Disability (YLDs), one of several metrics used to assess disease impact on humans.

Despite the prevalence and impact of low back pain, modern medicine has utterly failed to treat and prevent it. Pain pills and analgesics remain the primary go-to. While surgery should be a last-ditch, Hail Mary, buzzer shot from half court strategy, it is shockingly common, unethically expensive, and dismally ineffective.

The Institute of Medicine (IOM), the National Institute of Health (NIH), and the World Health Organization (WHO) all agree on the universal and urgent need for more effective methods of treatment for low back pain as well as more cost-effective ways of providing them.

While the need for change is worldwide, Americans get the worst of it, with back surgery rates at least 40% higher than any other country, and five times as high as our neighbors across the pond. Despite the inefficacy of back surgery, people continue to patronize and prolong its economic viability. And economically viable it is! If you want to understand a thing, all you need to do is follow the money. Low back pain (LBP) has a major economic impact in the United States, with total costs related to this condition exceeding $100 billion per year. Somebody, somewhere, is getting filthy rich off the backs of people in pain.

These costs are increasing over time. Indeed, the average cost of spinal fusions increased from $24,676 in 1998 to $81,960 in 2008! That's nearly 800% more than the increase in the U.S. economy in the same time period.[1]

With these kinds of numbers, back pain is big business. Why solve a problem with such massive bankroll? People are greedy. No surprise there. So, the better question is: Why do we continue to waste our precious time and resources on treatment that not only doesn't work but often comes with serious side effects? The short answer is: It just feels... normal. We've literally never known anything different. So we accept it. But now we need to make it un-normal. We need to see the light. Let's illuminate things with a quick history lesson.

---

[1] "The U.S. economy to 2008: a decade of continued growth." https://www.bls.gov/opub/mlr/1999/11/art2full.pdf. Accessed 19 Aug. 2020.

How did this become so normal? If we can put a man on the moon, if we can cure polio, if we can transplant a human heart — why on earth (or even space) can we not successfully treat back pain? Well, we can. The reason it seems like we cannot is because we are living inside the convoluted box that is modern medicine. Just like casinos deliberately make their floor plans hard to escape and thus encourage more gambling, the medical world keeps its denizens in a maze that few escape. But where did this box come from? When did medicine become modern? Some of its origins are malicious, with corruption, greed, and disregard for human life at the core. Some of it is truly no one's fault. Let's pop out the X-Acto knife, slice through the tape, and open this box.

The box is the product of a massive shift in politics, technology, economics, and cultural identity. Let's rewind the clock to get oriented...

The year is 1863. A particularly gruesome battle between the North and South has just ended: the Battle of Gettysburg. In its aftermath, over 50,000 casualties are counted. Unfortunately for the wounded, the X-ray would not be discovered until 1895, nor would penicillin be discovered until 1928. Indeed, the entire microscopic world of bacteria was only just being studied by Louis Pasteur. That meant most soldiers who survived the battlefields, bullets, and bayonets would soon die or become permanently crippled due to crude amputations, poor sterilization, and lack of antibiotics. But you didn't have to fight in an infamous civil war battle to be in danger. The typical American family lived under constant threat of diseases like tuberculosis and influenza. Even diarrhea was a life-threatening condition! Clearly, medicine was not the technological marvel that it is today. Given the dire circumstances, it is not hard to see why advancements in medical technology were joyously received by our great-great-grandparents.

Besides new technologies, medical ethics were also maturing. With its inception in 1849, the American Medical Association's first task was to expose and dispel the quackery that plagued medicine.[2] This was the dawn of a new era of professionalism in medicine. The AMA helped set minimum-competency requirements in education and training, established peer-reviewed research communities, and defined a standard of practice that allowed patients to receive similar care wherever they went. A day had finally arrived where most licensed doctors could be trusted to provide the best possible care!

Let's pause. Advancements in medical science. Good. Advancements in medical ethics. Great. Where did things go awry? This is the complicated part, but we'll try to keep it simple.

On an individual level, Americans originally had a strong sense of self-reliance and acceptance of suffering and death. The reason for this is fairly obvious: They were constantly surrounded by it! And unlike today, there were no mass-produced painkillers like Tylenol, nor were there 24/7 urgent care centers located on every other block. Instead of blind adherence to prescriptions and medical procedures, 19th century Americans had to rely on traditional

---

[2] "AMA history | American Medical Association." 20 Nov. 2018, https://www.ama-assn.org/about/ama-history/ama-history. Accessed 19 Aug. 2020.

Chapter 1: Modern Medicine's Failure to Address Low Back Pain

wisdom to stay strong, avoid illness, and recover as best as possible. Though frequently subject to superstition, tradition nonetheless guided innumerable generations in nutrition, exercise, parenthood, illness, recovery, and social relationships.

From a modern-day understanding of pain science, this sense of self-reliance and acceptance is extremely powerful in minimizing both the short- and long-term effects of pain and suffering.[3] It actually stimulates the immune system and speeds recovery in a way that all the vitamin C and Tylenol in the world cannot match. And we've all but lost it! Our forebears also had an understanding that health could not be expedited or taken in pill form. They understood that it consisted of a balance of rest, work, food, and relationships. Today? We don't just have drive-thru fast food; we have drive-thru pharmacies.

On a systemic level, medicine peaked when it solved biomedical problems according to the biomedical model. The biomedical model essentially comes from Descartes' philosophy of reductionism. It proposes that the best way to solve a problem is to break it down into the smallest possible pieces. This works well when the problems have a single source. For example, isolating the polio virus made it possible to create a vaccine. Thanks to reductionism and the biomedical model, polio (and many other viral/bacterial illnesses) are now eradicated!

Unfortunately, most of the diseases that we face now come not from individual viruses or bacteria but instead from systemic flaws in our lifestyle. For example, type 2 diabetes is not a disease that you could catch if someone sneezed on you. Instead, it is a complex disorganization of hormones and metabolic factors that allows toxic levels of sugar to accumulate in the blood. It results from lifestyle factors such as excessive consumption of sugars and sedentary behavior. While the biomedical model has isolated blood sugar imbalance as the problem and insulin as the treatment, it is only a temporary bandage, not a cure. Just as there is no vaccine to cure diabetes, there is no single drug, injection, or surgery that cures back pain. It is a systemic problem with multiple contributing lifestyle factors.

Magnetic resonance imaging, better known as MRI, is an incredible imaging technology first used in 1977. The MRI may be able to show deviations from the norm, such as a protruding L4-L5 disc. Then, doctors may even be able to surgically treat that segment in isolation, but it rarely solves the whole problem, and thus millions of people continue to suffer with back pain even after surgery. Although the biomedical model initially helped to accelerate medical technology and save lives, in the past 50 years it has slowed the medical community from treating conditions like low back pain successfully.

If you're feeling a tiny bit confused, some problems are isolated and an isolated solution can solve them (like polio), while others, like low back pain, are systemic and require systemic change to fix them. Pills, injections, surgeries, and anything that attempts to identify and treat a single issue fall short of the systemic nature of low back pain.

---

[3] "AMA history | American Medical Association." 20 Nov. 2018, https://www.ama-assn.org/about/ama-history/ama-history. Accessed 19 Aug. 2020.

Because of inefficacy of the isolated solutions strategy, a new paradigm called the biopsychosocial model has begun to shape medical research and treatment. It takes into account complicated human behavioral and lifestyle factors.[4] Unfortunately, it is hard to teach an old dog new tricks. The biomedical model is so entrenched in medical education, procedure, and even billing/insurance, that it will be decades before major changes occur. Even then, it will be slow going. Why? Because those who have the greatest ability to change it are also the ones who profit the most from it. If you make money off sick people, why would you be motivated to actually help them not be sick? Well, I could think of ten reasons off the top of my head (and I'm sure you could think of ten more), but the way you and I think is quite different from that type of person.

How is it that this system became so entrenched? After the Second World War, the U.S. government grew in size as well as connection to large industrial and commercial companies. The reason was simple: While under threat of a common enemy, everybody pulled together to produce goods and services for the war effort. Companies that previously had no government affiliation whatsoever were now highly connected to public policy. All of that cohesiveness and shared purpose allowed for great prosperity.

Thus, post-war America was a place of unprecedented optimism and trust. However, it also allowed a blurring of the lines between the public and private sectors. This set the stage for pharmaceutical and medical lobbyists to exert significant influence on the government. As a massive industry with powerful government ties, it is too easy for corrupt corporate leaders and politicians to take advantage of health consumers, and too hard for good-hearted medical professionals and legislators to actualize reform.

Is this picture starting to sound pretty bleak? Fear not! The U.S. is still a land of opportunity, and it is not difficult to escape the corporate medical authority and move into a new season of health. It may not happen on a grand scale for the whole population, but if you are reading this, know that it is within your power individually to get better. And that is the purpose of this book: to get you better.

So, how do we get better? Well, what if back pain was simply a commonsense problem with a commonsense solution? To truly cure low back pain requires an understanding of a few simple truths about how our bodies work and what environments we choose to occupy. The simple truths are that we do better when we feel safe than when we feel like we are in imminent danger. However, in our attempts to pursue safety, stability, and comfort, we've wound up in more danger than ever.

It's not hard for most people in pain to realize that their bodies need to heal. They may not be sure WHAT they need to heal from, but they know they need to heal. It is nearly impossible for our bodies to heal if they sense imminent danger. When we sense imminent danger, we tend to create an inflammatory response that amplifies and extends our experience of pain.

---

4 "The Continuing and Growing Epidemic of … - NCBI - NIH." https://www.ncbi.nlm.nih.gov/pmc/articles/PMC4939568/. Accessed 19 Aug. 2020.

Chapter 1: Modern Medicine's Failure to Address Low Back Pain

Thus, to get at the heart of pain, we have to get at the heart of inflammation. And to get at the heart of inflammation, we have to figure out how to restore a sense of safety in a dangerous world.

Read on to learn how to move past the red tape of the medical industry, get the best of modern and traditional medicine, and be on your way to an incredible, pain-free life.

For All Its Naughtiness, Sometimes Modern Medicine Is Nice...

Let's say you decide to go out and hang Christmas lights yourself (never smart). You slip off the ladder and fall 15 feet to the ground. You're hurt pretty bad (sorry, this is morbid, but bear with us!) and you're rushed to the hospital in an ambulance. You are losing blood, but the doctors are able to save you through a blood transfusion. They prevent infection through medications that if you had not taken, you would have died. Without the advances in modern medicine in the last 50 years, you would have been dead. But thanks to our medical system, you are alive and well (if only ladders hadn't been invented, you would have been totally fine!). Our medical system is really good when it comes to helping people not die.

But — it is woefully inept at keeping people healthy.

Yet, many people in our society today are reliant on the medical system to keep them healthy. It's as if there is a sense of entitlement to be taken care of because we pay for health insurance.

We don't do this with our cars, but we do it with our bodies. We want our car insurance to come into play if we are in an accident. Yet we wouldn't expect our car insurance to pay for oil changes, tire rotations, or serpentine belt replacements.

In fact, you probably budget money each month for routine car maintenance (or you just put it on a credit card).

It's the same with our bodies. Except in this case, we only get one body our entire life.

So, with that "one body," it's essential for you to learn and study the operator's manual. It's essential to care for it well, perform routine maintenance, and figure out the root cause of problems going on (like low back pain), instead of masking symptoms with pills, injections, manipulations, or surgeries.

We want to put you in the driver's seat for your health (or the passenger seat so you can better reach the operator's manual in the glove compartment...).

Chapter 2: The Inflammastories

A collection of tales halfway between analogy and analgesic

One of the greatest obstacles between you and solving your back pain is the massive knowledge gap between you and the medical community. To bridge this gap with minimal difficulty, we've written the following analogies to give you a remarkably profound level of physiological understanding without any technical medical training. They are purposefully a little goofy, hopefully entertaining, and will serve as a broad backdrop for your unique journey.

We start with Bodville, the most in-depth of the analogies, which get progressively simpler from there.

Bodville, USA

Welcome to the small town of Bodville. In Bodville, there are two little shops. One is Cool Hound Luke's Pet Shop, the other, Murphy's Lawn Care Emporium. Both businesses are exposed to similar criminal activity from the local gang leader, Danger Dan. Danger Dan is a disgruntled man who feels he should have been Junior Prom King and is forever jealous of the man who robbed him of the coveted title. That man is Safety Steve, who is now Mayor of Bodville. Safety Steve tries to keep things mellow, but Danger Dan loves to stir up trouble. However, Danger Dan is more bark than bite. He's only caused real harm a handful of times, and that was when his cousin, Damage Dom, went with him. Mayor Steve's right-hand men are Repair Rick and Maintenance Mick. Repair Rick is the best in the business and can fix almost anything, but he is rarely seen in public. Usually it's just Maintenance Mick who makes rounds and keeps Bodville running smoothly.

Cool Hound Luke's Pet Shop

At Cool Hound Luke's, all employees are trained to respond to threatening situations with a calm, cool head. The owner, Luke Pneuman, has seen his fair share of criminals and isn't intimidated easily. Like most businesses in the area, Luke's has a few Danger Alarms set up to alert them if Dan comes around. Since he rarely does more than yell obscenities and empty threats, they only activate the emergency response system when there is true suspicious activity. Most of the time, they just request a single patrol to check things out. None of the employees have ever seen a dangerous situation get out of hand, and they have no reason to believe it ever will. Every once in a great while, Danger Dan and Damage Dom show up together and break a few windows, but when this happens, Safety Steve sends Repair Rick to the rescue, and all is well. They have a great relationship with the city board and local authorities. Luke votes for Safety Steve every year.

Murphy's Lawn Care Emporium

At Murphy's, it seems like anything that could go wrong does go wrong. During their grand opening, Danger Dan and his cronies broke in and stole Mr. Murphy's flagship fleet of Don Jeer Tractors. They proceeded to joyride through town, leaving traumatized civilians and perfectly manicured hedges in their wake. Mr. Murphy is now so paranoid about being robbed that he rarely goes home, choosing instead to sleep in one of the reclining lawn chairs on display. In fact, Mr. Murphy no longer trusts local authorities to respond to his hourly calls for help. Instead, he has privately contracted Inflammatory Fred's Superfluous Security Syndicate. It is not uncommon to see a Black Hawk Helicopter descend and missile strike a squirrel scuttling around the roof. Of course, this has the unfortunate tendency of blowing up half the property. By the time Murphy has paid for all the repairs and incinerated merchandise, the cost is far greater than anything Danger Dan has ever done. Despite multiple warnings from his accountant, Mr. Murphy prefers the sense of control that self-sabotage gives him. We won't even get into the troubles of Mr. and Mrs. Murphy's marriage!

Maintenance Mick rarely steps foot in Murphy's anymore, as Murphy now employs several blind Doberman shepherds as handymen. Like the pet store nearby, Murphy also has Danger Alarms set up. However, Murphy has reprogrammed them to go off any time they sense Dan within a 20-mile radius. Since Bodville is only a small town, they are almost constantly going off! Strangely, Murphy has actually been considering supporting Danger Dan as the new mayor of Bodville.

The Allegory

Bodville	Your whole body!
Safety Steve	Representative of the body's amazing ability to coordinate multiple systems, including our nervous system and immune system, to keep us healthy and maintain homeostasis.
Maintenance Mick	Representative of low-level immune system activity, clearing out daily metabolic waste products from muscles used to walk around, and things like preventing infections from small amounts of germs on door handles.
Repair Rick	Representative of high-level immune system activity, such as fever or major swelling around a broken ankle.
Danger Dan	Danger Dan: Representative of all the threats that our bodies face — what we perceive to be dangerous.
Damage Dom	Representative of actual injuries sustained to our bodies.

Bodville, you have a body! It's where you live. It's where you sleep. It is a gift and also a tool. Wherever you go, there it will be also. It is not just anywhere USA, but anywhere in the universe! It is the only physical thing you are guaranteed to have from the moment you're born until your very last breath. And it is the single greatest place to invest if you want to make an impact on the world around you and the people you love.

No matter where you go with your body, you will be exposed to danger. There is no safety bubble for you to stay in. Yet, built right into your body, right into your genetic code, is everything you need to be safe in a dangerous world. So, who has more power in your body: Danger Dan or Safety Steve? Who do you want to have more power?

Safety Steve represents our perception of security, stability, and, you guessed it, safety.

Danger Dan represents our perception of threat — what we perceive can cause us harm.

Damage Dom represents actual harm done to our bodies. In a world where everything made perfect sense, they would be inseparable. But our world doesn't always make perfect sense, and they often are separate.

A Story From Dr. Erik's Childhood

How does Danger Dan sabotage us?

When I was a little kid, I loved cute, fuzzy animals. I mean, I still do. Does anybody not? One year, I begged my parents to let me get a few pet mice. Mom said no, and on Christmas morning, I unwrapped a Beanie Baby mouse from Santa while my mom sported a rueful grin. Next, my dad said my brother and I had a shared present that was in the basement. Guess what it was? Rueful means simultaneous sorrow and humor. If there is a word that means simultaneous surprise and rage, that was the next expression my mom wore. Because in the basement were some very cute, very alive, pet mice.

So, we had these mice, and soon they got busy making more mice. The original mice were all pretty nice, but a few of their offspring turned out to be little mouse monsters. Mousters?

One day, while I was reaching into their cage to change the water, a particularly nasty black mouse that we called Psyches (because he was psychotic) bit my finger. It didn't even pierce the skin, but the surprise was enough for me to jerk my hand out of the cage with all the power of a sprinter off the gun. The problem is that the opening to the cage was pretty small, and my wrist caught the edge of the opening, which resulted in the entire cage being flung across the room as well as a large bloody gash on my forearm.

Meanwhile, my poor pet mice endured something similar to the meteor that killed the dinosaurs hitting their little mouse world. Worst of all, Psyches got out. True to his nature, his interest was not in freedom per se, but in causing us prolonged pain and suffering. Escape to the wild world beyond he did not. Remain in our house and scream across the floor when we had company over he did.

So, in this little story, Danger Dan got the best of me. I reacted to a tiny mouse nibble like my head was in the mouth of a lion. Was Damage Dom in that little nibble? Not really. Ironically, the true threat of damage was in my reaction, but I had no sense of danger about such a reaction.

In the same way, professional emergency response teams are trained to see the danger of panic because of its high propensity for real damage. The more you understand about Damage Dom, the less you will react to Danger Dan.

Chapter 2: The Inflammastories

Maintenance Mick, Repair Rick, and Inflammatory Fred's Superfluous Security Syndicate

Mick represents the day-to-day action of a functional immune system, while Rick represents a major action of a functional immune system in response to something seriously threatening.

Mick is present in our bodies 24/7. He deals with tons of little pathogens that we inhale, drink, eat, and touch, as well as microtears in our muscles, joints, and connective tissues from daily movement and exercise, even the effects of brief exposure to UV light from the sun.

Rick goes into action for the big stuff. He's the reason we get a fever when we're trying to fend off a flu, or the reason our ankle swells up like a balloon after a massive sprain.

Inflammatory Fred's represents a dysfunctional immune system response. It is the same system, so it has the same effects — things like increased nerve sensitivity, swelling, warmth, and redness — but totally excessive and misguided. Our patients are often amazed to learn that inflammation does not mean an actual injury exists. But this is not actually groundbreaking. Think about allergies. What is an allergy but a dysfunctionally excessive immune response? I have the misfortune of being allergic to most things on the planet. I'm serious.

Murphy's or Luke's?

If Bodville represents your body, Cool Hound Luke's and Murphy's represent two potential versions of the same immune system.

Murphy's represents the type of person who perceives great danger, has terrible perception of true damage, and has very little confidence in their body's ability to heal. Murphy's could be a person who was in a traumatic car accident 20 years ago that still feels like it was yesterday. Most of the current pain and inflammatory symptoms are the result of a heightened sense of danger and dysfunctional immune response, as opposed to immediate physical injury.

Cool Hound Luke's represents the type of person who knows not to panic every time they see danger. Even when they are injured, they get an accurate assessment of the damage and determine the best possible pathway to healing. Even when this type of person gets into a terrible car accident and seriously ruptures a spinal disc, they keep their thoughts and feelings collected and accept the situation for what it is. They gather several expert opinions, weigh it against their own knowledge, needs, and goals, and make an estimate about how long they will need to fully heal. Then they do what's necessary to put their body in the best possible environment to heal. They don't worry about all the things that could go wrong, and they write down the questions and unknowns that arise along the journey to deal with when most appropriate.

In the next part of the book, we will talk in-depth about the exact plan and principles you need in place in your life to be less like Murphy's and more like Luke's.

Boddington Castle

Imagine a medieval castle. Ten bucks says you are now picturing the Disney castle. This castle has a king, soldiers, and villagers. Currently, there is peace throughout the land. The villagers are safe and going about their daily business. The builders are building. The farmers are farming. The artists are... arting, er, painting. The King is tweeting about "Saturday Night Live," and the soldiers are resting up, polishing their armor, and helping to deal with minor squabbles between villagers. But then one day, looming on the far-off hillside, an invading army approaches. Village life changes. The villagers go into lockdown inside the castle walls. The soldiers mobilize to defensive positions. Even the King takes action, albeit still via Twitter.

As a result, the village is no longer occupied with becoming a larger, more beautiful place. Instead, it uses all of its resources for survival. If the invading army is soon defeated, life will pretty much go back to normal. The villagers will come out from lockdown and begin making repairs to the castle and helping the soldiers mend up. But what if the invading army isn't defeated right away? What if a state of battle and emergency stretches from days into weeks into months?

Eventually, the soldiers will get worn out, or worse! As a last-ditch effort to defend the castle, the villagers themselves may have to fight. Even the artists. As you can imagine, the castle may not have much longer to survive in this dire state when a bunch of guys with paintbrushes are going up against steel and swords.

In this analogy, the castle is your body. During times of peace and health, your body has many different types of cells performing different roles, much like the villagers and their various vocations. Just as the villagers are able to grow and improve the castle, so you are able to grow smarter, stronger, and enjoy just being alive. The soldiers represent your immune system. During times of relative health, they are mostly there to deal with minor stuff.

Now, as for the invading army, that can be any number of threats to your body. It could be a serious viral infection. Or it could be a major musculoskeletal injury like a broken bone. You should have more than enough bodily resources to defend against illness and injury. Once the threat is gone, lots of cells in your body should go to work helping you rest, heal and recover. Once that's over, they can go back to helping you grow and fulfill your lifelong dream of becoming a traveling bubblegum salesman. However, if the battle is long enough, your immune system may become depleted of its resources. At that point, the body may have to start compromising its storehouses to prolong your survival. This is often what happens when we get stuck in a rut of chronic stress, pain, and inflammation. In other words, even when the invading army is gone, the body can be left in a state where it is so weak that it thinks it is still under attack.

Chapter 2: The Inflammastories

Life Is A Highway

How our body feels when we were kids is like that gorgeous section of the California 134 just before Glendale at 6 a.m. on a Sunday, with nothing but birds chirping and sunshine warming the hilltops across the valley. You could careen across six lanes and be totally safe. Not that you should. But you could.

The older you get, the closer you get towards Monday morning on the oldest section of the 5 (for those who have never dealt with California traffic, the I-5 is one of the worst highways in the country for traffic). And yes, multiple lanes are blocked due to accidents. If your car is an ailing Crown Victoria and you haven't had any coffee, the chances of you running into someone and causing the next lane blockage are high.

Most folks are worried that it's too late for their bodies to get them where they want to go. They're too old and too injured. They're up against the guardrail in life's highway. Now, it may not be possible to find six open lanes of freedom the way it was as a kid, but the good news is that you don't need all six lanes open to move at a comfortable speed. You just need one. So, what's that lane for you? Maybe it's nutrition, maybe it's healthy movement, or maybe it's understanding pain and inflammation through analogies like this one.

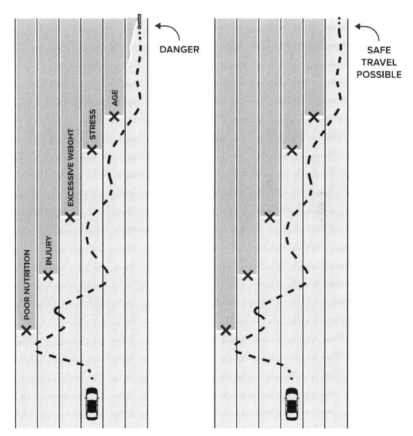

Sacred Ice Cream

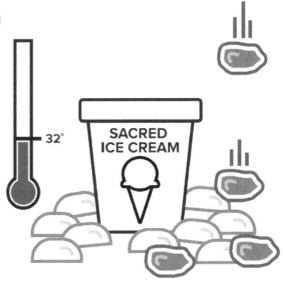

I know a lot of people who really, really like ice cream. Side note on ice cream: If you love it, make your own. Raw heavy cream, vanilla bean, a dab of maple syrup, and a machine you can buy on Amazon for 40 bucks will change your life. Side note over. So, let's say you have a cooler full of sacred ice cream that must make it to its destination. To get there, the ice cream must stay below 32 degrees. It could be below 32; it just cannot be above. Otherwise... it starts to melt! Of course, ice cream can melt a teeny-tiny bit at the top and still be fine. But if the whole carton is liquid... bad news.

So, in this hypothetical situation, ice cubes and hot coals are getting thrown into the cooler. Obviously, the hot coals put the ice cream in danger of melting, while the ice cubes protect it. Every time you do something for your body like getting good sleep, getting a massage, or eating anti-inflammatory foods, it's like throwing ice cubes in the cooler. Every time you sit at a desk for eight hours straight or chow down on French fries, it's like throwing in hot coals. You can get away with a few hot coals, but they need to be covered by ice cubes.

You may have a preexisting condition that is very difficult to solve, like rheumatoid arthritis or scoliosis, and this makes your coolers warmer to begin with (kind of like having a lid that doesn't quite close all the way). But fear not! You are not doomed. If the ice cream doesn't melt, you get to live a full, happy life. This just means you need to get as many ice-cubes in the cooler as you can — enough to keep the temperature below 32.

You may be bitter or frustrated that other people have a colder temperature to begin with, but what's the point in comparing yourself to others? The important reality to focus on is that you can still be happy and healthy. Many of the low back pain patients we work with have scoliosis, which we will cover in a later chapter. Scoliosis tends to make people more sensitive to pain. It's like starting with a cooler that has a lid that will never close all the way. It's tougher to keep cool, but not impossible. Here's the cool thing: Even with significant cases of scoliosis, we've seen patients add enough ice cubes (through the plan and principles laid out later in this book) to live a pain-free, active life. We may not have been able to change the way your cooler closes, but we can add enough ice cubes to bring the sacred ice cream under 32 degrees.

Chapter 2: The Inflammastories

Cup O' Inflammation

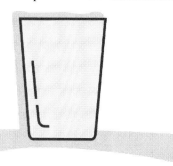

Similar but simpler than the cooler analogy above is what we call Cup O' Inflammation. If the cup doesn't overflow, life is good. It could be half-empty. If you're an optimist, it could be half-full. It could be totally empty. It could be right at the brim. If it doesn't spill over, no symptoms of pain, weakness, stiffness, or lack of performance are experienced. Things like congenital abnormalities or permanent wear and tear (think osteoarthritis) can raise the water level, but need not make the cup spill over. What most often makes these cups spill over are things like brutally tense muscles, un-lubricated joints, lack of sleep, poor nutrition, general under-use muscle loss, and stress neural tension. In other words, there are a lot of very solvable problems that should be taken care of before being discouraged about what an MRI said about your bone-on-bone knees or lumbar stenosis!

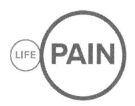

Life and Pain

This visual is all about perspective. As humans, we love to live! But a lot of stuff can get in the way of living, and our lives can seem very small. In the famous words of Henry David Thoreau, "The mass of men lead lives of quiet desperation." The less connected and purposeful we feel, the more our senses are tuned to discomfort, frustration, bitterness, and ultimately, pain. In turn, a downward spiral compounds the phenomenon. It's hard to "stop and smell the roses" when your back pain prevents you from getting out into your yard to begin with!

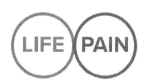

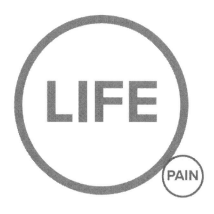

Just because this stuff has to do with attitude and perspective doesn't mean it isn't real. Physiologically, getting stuck in a negative mindset actually pushes us into what is technically called the sympathetic division of the autonomic nervous system, what you may have heard of as the "fight-or-flight" response. This should not be underestimated! We believe there is always more going for you than against you. We believe there is always more that you can do than you cannot do. By playing to your strengths, you can grow the green circle of life to utterly dwarf the red circle of pain.

The Nonlinear Path

We humans like things simple, and what could be simpler than a straight line? When it comes to healing, our expectation is often that each stage of healing will occur consistently and sequentially. Yet, our true healing journeys are better represented in the second circle. Depending on where we start, we may spend longer in some phases than others. We may even find that sometimes things get worse before they get better. On your own, this process can be confusing at best and outright soul-crushing at worst. Fortunately, we have walked through this journey ourselves as well as with thousands of clients, so we have enough perspective to help you navigate your body's unique path while remaining encouraged, hopeful, and confident you are going in the right direction.

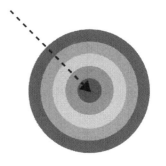

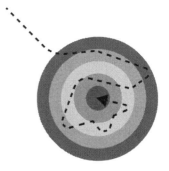

Skill vs. Material

The best chefs in the world not only possess amazing culinary skill but also have access to ingredients that your local Sprouts can only dream of, not to mention state-of-the-art kitchens. Still, imagine a Michelin-starred chef in your kitchen, using your knives, your little stove, and whatever ingredients they can find in your cupboards. Chances are they could still make something mouthwatering! Conversely, even the most average (is "most average" an oxymoron?) home chef could construct a delicious, fresh salad if they got to pick the tomatoes and greens from a sunny Tuscan farm, drizzle with just-pressed olive oil, and garnish with aged Parmesan cheese.

Through this book, we will talk about building better raw materials into your body as well as increasing skill in using your body. While some raw material is a matter of genetics, there is a ton that can be done over time to obtain "better ingredients." We build better raw materials by

Chapter 2: The Inflammastories

improving what food we put into our bodies, strengthening muscles and bones, lubricating joints, and mobilizing nerves. We increase our skill by surrounding ourselves with experts, deliberately practicing movement patterns, and challenging our coordination.

Sometimes we sell ourselves short because we were born with conditions like asthma or scoliosis, because we currently have conditions like diabetes or even cancer, or simply because we feel like we are over the hill in age and it's too late to get healthy. We feel like we don't have the raw material to make any progress. The first good news is that virtually any person who is warm and breathing can drastically change what they're made of by changing what they eat and using their bodies right where they are. The even better news is that there is NO LIMIT to improving in skill. With the right coaching and consistent discipline, you can go from disabled or missing out to vibrantly living.

Butch Cartilage and the Trust Fund Kid

Imagine a trust fund kid. Reckless. Irresponsible. Pretty much able to get away with murder because he can always pay someone off from his sizeable bank account. This is what our bodies are like when we're young. We have enough cushion in our joints to escape from terrible movement faults, like always bending from your back when you reach forward to grab a toy off the ground or allowing your head to jut forward while you text. We can even get away with eating toxic foods and poor sleep with minimal consequence (in the moment). But nobody respects the trust fund kid.

Contrast this kid with a blue-collar worker who begins budgeting, saving, and investing wisely. Although this person cannot do exorbitant things with their money, they can live a very good, very full life.

Now, what if we were talking about joint cartilage instead of money? The problem for most folks is that their perspective on age-related changes in their bodies is in reference to when they were kids. Trust fund kids. Just because you cannot be reckless and irresponsible with your body does not mean you cannot live fully and do all the things you want to do. Plenty of people with spines and knees that are bone-on-bone are climbing mountains. But they are also saving, budgeting, and investing their health dollars, figuratively and literally. And that's respectable in a way that rash spending can never be.

Bottom line: It would be nice to have millions of dollars of joint cartilage between your bones. But you can get by just fine on a few thousand.

Chapter 3: Turning Pain Science Into Plain Science

Since infancy, we learn that our world can hurt us. We learn that we can skin knees, bump heads, and even feel painful tears when we are left out or angry. We learn that some of our hurts heal while others linger. Sometimes we even experience pain so profoundly that it alters the course of our lives. Chances are you know someone whose pain led them to drastic choices, like leaving a job, a marriage, or even their religion. You probably know even more people who have pursued risky surgeries or developed dependencies to medications aimed at reducing pain. Yet, despite its ubiquity, few understand what pain actually is. Pain science is simply the science of understanding pain — the objective study of what it is, and what it is not. But before we get into that, what do you think it is?

Take a moment and try to define it. Is it a feeling? Is it a signal? Is it physical? Emotional? Is it good? Bad? Helpful or harmful?

At a low back pain workshop we hosted, we asked folks why they had back pain. Here were a few of their responses:

"It's because I have degenerative discs," one lady piped up.

"My back hurts because my family has bad backs," said another gentleman.

A man in his mid-50s replied, "I was in a car accident five years ago, and it's never been the same."

Raising her hand, a lady in the back confessed, "I have a pinched nerve."

"Because I'M OLD!" roared a middle-aged man who definitely was not that old.

So, which answer is correct? Pain is remarkably hard to put in a box. It's complex. It's often many things at once. So, let's try to take things one at a time. To motivate you to keep reading, know that research indicates the more you understand about pain, the less pain you will have![5]

---

5   "Pain is Weird: A Volatile, Misleading Sensation - Pain Science." 26 Aug. 2018, https://www.painscience.com/articles/pain-is-weird.php. Accessed 27 Sep. 2018.

What each person in our workshop was expressing was not necessarily what caused their pain, but what caused them to feel threatened. It was the thing that caused them to feel the opposite of safety. For one person, they felt threatened by their knowledge of family members with similar pain. For another, they felt threatened by the process of aging. For another, it was an image they had in their head of a big nerve pinched between vertebrae, red and swollen like a finger pinched in a door frame. Each person in the workshop had a unique set of life experiences, prior knowledge, and personality that made certain things stand out as threatening. What they had in common was a connection between the sensations from their backs with the phenomenon of pain.

"But wait," you might be thinking, "don't I have pain because I have an injury? It sounds like you're saying that my pain is all in my head, or my attitude, or personality… or something! But I know my back is injured because an MRI showed a bulging disc!" This is a totally fair, very common response when introduced to pain science.

The assumption is that pain and bodily damage correlate on a direct 1:1 ratio. More pain equals more damage, and more damage equals more pain. Therefore, if one feels a lot of pain, there must be a lot of damage. Furthermore, if one is to get out of pain, one must simply heal or fix the damaged body part. It is for this reason that the prospect of surgery is so often enticing. We like the idea that a damaged body part simply needs to be undamaged in order to get relief.

To be fair, this assumption is not a ridiculous idea. It comes from the understanding of our bodies that we develop as kids, when we are fairly healthy. It is often reinforced by the knowledge we are taught in schools and in doctor's offices. Then, it is repeated by our friends and throughout our culture and language, solidifying it in our subconscious as absolute truth.

But it is not. What we experienced as healthy kids was an ideal healing response. After falling off a bike and skinning our knees, we saw the tissue damage with our eyes. Then we felt the pain. Then, a few weeks later, when the cut was all gone and new skin covered the wound, we felt no pain. Now ask yourself, if you were simply experiencing an ideal healing response, wouldn't you feel better by now? As a matter of fact, nearly all body tissues should finish their healing process within three months. If it has been longer than three months, what is the deal?

Here's the deal: Either you have a healing problem with your actual tissues, or you have a communication problem in your neuro-immune system, or both. Towards the end of this book, we will introduce you to the 12 Village Principles. Most folks who follow these 12 principles should provide their bodies with everything necessary for tissue healing, including things like the right nutrition for rebuilding damaged-tissue. Additionally, the very next chapter will cover all sorts of commonly damaged tissues like sciatic nerves, discs, and so on. However, all the tissue healing in the world won't matter if the communication problem persists. In fact, many folks with no tissue damage whatsoever still experience debilitating pain.

Chapter 3: Turning Pain Science Into Plain Science

So, if you're like most folks with low back pain: "What we've got here is a failure to communicate!"

The Sensation-Threat-Danger-Alarm-Pain-Action System

We made up the name, but it's pretty accurate.

What is sensation?

Before pain, before threats, before alarms, we simply have sensation. At the most basic level, sensation is information that your body gathers about your environment as well as your own body. It is information about temperature, physical pressure, chemical reactions, and all sorts of things. It helps you to live in your body and navigate your environment safely and enjoyably.

Sensation begins at a structure called the nerve receptor. Nerve receptors usually get their name from the scientist who discovered them, such as Meisner, Merkel, and Pacini, but don't worry, there is no quiz on this at the end of the chapter. We have different nerve receptors for different types of sensations. For example, your tongue has pressure receptors that can feel the texture of your food, while chemical receptors are responsible for the actual taste.

Speaking of tastes, it is common knowledge that the same food can taste delicious to one person and disgusting to another. We often say that we "have different tastes." In fact, we not only apply this concept to the taste of food, but even to things like taste in music, film, clothing, even career and vocation. Additionally, the same food that "hits the spot" one day may make you nauseous the next day. Does this mean the nerve receptors changed from day to day or person to person? More likely, there is something else occurring to affect how that sensation is perceived. We'll get to that later, as well as how it is paramount in solving chronic pain.

For now, just know that sensation begins with nerve receptors, and that there is no single nerve receptor that is responsible for pain. Because pain is not in and of itself a sensation in the same way that pressure, temperature, chemicals, stretch, vibration, etc. are.

Still, while there is no specific nerve receptor for pain, there is indeed an array of receptors for nociception, or danger. At this point, pain and danger might sound like the same thing, but they are not. So be advised: Do not confuse what we are about to talk about regarding danger as though it was synonymous with pain. Deal? Thanks.

Nociceptors exist to help us determine when a sensation goes from being safe to being dangerous. Imagine you are drawing a bath and you want it to be that perfect temperature that is wonderfully hot but not scalding. Have you ever fiddled back and forth with the faucet knob between lukewarm and boiling? It was the nociceptors in the skin of your finger that helped figure out how hot you could get your water before being in danger of getting burned. Contrast the experience of testing the water with your finger to accidentally pouring boiling water on yourself while draining a big pot of spaghetti (obviously carbs are dangerous in multiple ways). In that situation, your experience went beyond danger and into the realm of pain.

But for now let's stay in the realm of danger and nocception. Nociceptors are scattered amongst other nerve receptors (Merkel, Pacinian, etc.), yet they send signals to the brain a little differently. All nerve receptors require a certain amount of stimulation before sending a signal all the way to the brain. Without sufficient stimulation to the receptor, nothing is felt. This concept is usually described as "all or nothing." It is similar to the threshold for freezing. Water at 100 degrees Fahrenheit and water at 33 degrees Fahrenheit are both perfectly liquid; the water that is 1 degree away from freezing is no more frozen than the water that is 77 degrees away from freezing. Like the sending of a nerve impulse (known as an action potential), the change of water from liquid to solid is also an all-or-nothing phenomenon.

The way that nociceptors behave differently from other nerve receptors is that they transmit their signals more quickly to the brain. This is a great protective quality when the body is healthy. It means that your brain can perceive a threat and modify your behavior before you

What If You Didn't Feel Pain?

As a side note, imagine what it would be like if your nociceptors didn't work. Imagine the damage your body could incur from burns and cuts to your hands and feet. This is the reality for folks with diabetic neuropathy and other similar conditions. While you may wish that sometimes your nerves didn't work (and in fact there are even surgeries to cut off nerves entirely), they are truly there for your safety and longevity.

even realize what you are feeling. Have you ever almost stepped on something sharp? If you pay close attention, you'll realize that by the time you felt anything, your foot was already a foot in the air, totally recoiled and away from the dangerous sharp object.

Back to the idea of freezing water: Did you know that adding salt actually changes the temperature necessary to change from liquid to solid? It's still all or nothing; the water is either frozen or it's liquid. But the temperature at which that all-or-nothing change happens is different. Similarly, the body can add certain chemicals and compounds to the presence of nerve receptors to lower the threshold of stimulation necessary to create a signal that reaches the brain.

This is called peripheral sensitization. If you have ever gotten a sunburn, you know how excruciating a shower can be, even if the water is only lukewarm. The reason your danger threshold was lowered was because of the presence of pro-inflammatory compounds like cytokines and histamines released around your skin. The purpose of this is to help you stay extra safe while your tissues are healing. Other aspects of the healing inflammatory response include swelling from the presence of extra blood flow. This extra blood flow is necessary to clear out damaged cells and bring in brand-new building materials. While nobody likes the extra sensitivity and swelling, we can all be grateful our bodies are so clever at staying safe and repairing themselves when damaged.

Of course, no discussion about peripheral nerves is complete without mentioning the dorsal root ganglion, or DRG. The DRG is a sort of gate-way between the peripheral neuron and the spinal cord. Its role is to regulate the signals that the brain receives, either amplifying or diminishing them. As you've probably already guessed, it can play a big role in increasing the types of sensations you're trying to get relief from. This is both because of the way it modifies signals passing through and because the DRG itself can generate danger alarms that reach the brain. Because of their locations on the spinal column, certain spinal movements or positions can provoke the DRGs into their own unique alarm state. That's a good thing! The DRG are one of our first lines of danger-detection.

The next time you move into that certain position and feel a little danger explosion, be comforted that it is more likely to be a jumpy DRG than a severely damaged disc. In fact, it's not just the DRG that can make mountains out of molehills. Many of the weird, unpleasant things we feel stem from misbehaving nerves. If part of your back pain problem includes random itchiness, burning, zinging, or pins and needles, it's likely that peripheral nerves are involved.

But don't fret! Remember that everything we have discussed so far pertains more to threats and danger than to pain. So now, without further ado, the moment you've been waiting for...

Pain and the Brain

The organ with the single greatest influence on your pain problem is not located in your back muscles. It's not located in your spine. It's not even located in your peripheral nervous system. It's located in your head! It is the structures within the brain and nowhere else that are responsible for pain, and it is through understanding and addressing how the brain works that your pain problem will be truly solved. However, just because it is literally "in your head" does not mean that it is figuratively all in your head. To prove it, we're going to talk about one structure in the brain that has a particularly large impact on the interpretation of danger sensations as painful experiences, mention a few others, and then talk about how the brain physically manifests itself throughout the rest of your body through hormones and neurotransmitters.

So, what is this one structure in the brain that is responsible for so much suffering? Would you laugh if we said that it's an almond? What if we said it's Latin? Then we'd be talking about the amygdala. The amygdala is an almond-shaped area ("amygdala" comes from the Latin word for almond!) in the brain primarily responsible for connecting emotions, memories, and fear. Functioning perfectly, the amygdala is what helps us learn how to not be stupid. It helps children learn to not touch fire, not grab thistles (or step on them!), and stay away from pet dogs' mouths while they are eating. By permanently connecting negative emotions and memories of injury and insult, we are better able to avoid those injuries and insults in the future. Just like any other body part, the amygdala needs adequate rest. If overstimulated and under-rested, it can misfire.

This is exactly what happens in Post-Traumatic Stress Disorder, or PTSD. If you know anyone who suffers from PTSD, then you know how much hardship it can cause. Those who suffer are typically combat veterans, survivors of physical or psychological abuse, or victims of other catastrophic events like major car accidents or natural disasters. Symptoms include flashbacks, anxiety, apprehension, and a nervous system stuck in "danger mode."

Most chronic pain disorders behave similarly to PTSD, just on a smaller scale. While we have seen many patients with PTSD and chronic pain from major car accidents, we have also had patients with similar apprehensive behaviors and less severe chronic pain who simply "threw their back out" bending over to pick up something off the floor. While the latter typically do not need significant psychological care, their fearfulness of everyday tasks and body movements limits their freedom and enjoyment of life.

So, how is your amygdala? Is it serving you well and helping you avoid getting hurt? Or is it in overdrive, making you feel like any little movement or exercise could cause your back to implode in debilitating pain? Recall that the body behaves quite differently in safety mode and danger mode. Recall also that the body must spend most of its time in safety mode in order to thrive in daily life as well as have enough energy to weather occasional sickness and injury. If the amygdala begins interpreting too many situations as dangerous and linked to negative memories of injury, the body will remain in danger mode. As exhaustion sets in, it becomes harder and harder to feel safe again, establishing a downward spiral.

In this state, the amygdala begins to associate relatively safe movements and strains on the body as threatening. Let's compare again a healthy amygdala and an unhealthy amygdala with a common back pain complaint: pain while walking. When experiencing acute (short-term) back pain from a muscle strain, lots of normal activities can become painful, including something as simple as walking. The body is in an alarm state, and until it makes headway on healing, it more or less locks everything down so it can focus on essential immune stuff. Since the body is alarmed, it is important to give it space to do its thing and be patient while cellular regeneration occurs at a level that modern medicine hardly even understands. The amygdala temporarily associates walking with danger, but it is not a full-blown paranoia. It is more of a caution. So you walk cautiously, and as long as it gets a little better each day, no permanent danger is assigned by the amygdala to the activity of walking. But let's say there

Chapter 3: Turning Pain Science Into Plain Science

are a lot of other stresses in life, and let's say the immune system is already taxed due to poor nutrition and lifestyle habits. This amygdala may assign an excessive level of fear to walking.

If a healthy amygdala helps a child avoid stepping on thistles, an unhealthy amygdala causes panic anytime a child gets near a green field. If a healthy amygdala helps a child avoid burning his hands on a hot stove top, an unhealthy amygdala causes panic any time the child gets near a kitchen. If a healthy amygdala helps a person move gingerly for a few weeks after they strain a low back muscle while lifting improperly, an unhealthy amygdala creates a pain response years after the initial injury has healed every time they bend forward.

To summarize, the amygdala is the fear center of the brain. It closely links the emotional and memory centers of the brain with threatening experiences so that we can avoid danger in the future. When it malfunctions, it can assign excessive fear and avoidance to relatively safe activities and circumstances. The bottom line is that specific, situational cautions can help us avoid stupid injuries, while general panic does nothing but make a mess. Just because one time a black and white Siberian husky named Boris bit you when you hit it with a plastic yellow shovel (because you were three years old and your next-door neighbor Richie told you to and you didn't know better) doesn't mean you should be afraid of all dogs at all times, forever and ever. Not that that ever happened to me... Similarly, if your initials are B.J. and you have been training with us for several years and can jump a foot in the air while holding 110 pounds but are still afraid to do kettlebell swings because one time you hurt your back performing a deadlift, you just might have an amygdala in need of a little reassurance. B., if you are reading this, thanks for providing us with such a great example.

In addition to the amygdala, a few other key brain structures have been identified as playing a role in the experience of pain. In order to keep things simple for you, we won't delve too much into them. However, when you've got a problem, it's nice to have a place to point the finger. Giving these structures names can help you see that a vague statement like "It's all in your head" doesn't hold up. Blaming fingers ready? Off we go:

The hippocampus is at the top of the list. It might even be more accurate to read the above section on the amygdala with the hippocampus sort of tag-teaming to bring you pain, as it also plays a large role in memory and fear conditioning. Next on the list is the hypothalamus and thalamus, which modulate stress fight-or-flight responses. These can quicken your pulse, cause you to sweat, and mess with your body temperature, all frequent complaints of those with chronic low back pain. Then there is the sensory cortex, which is primarily responsible for discriminating between sensations. If your pain has moved and changed over time from one very specific area to several surrounding areas, there is a good chance your sensory cortex has changed your mental sensory map of your body. This change in the map can make us more sensitive to stimuli which normally would not be painful. If your pain makes it more difficult for you to concentrate, or rather the only thing on which you can concentrate is your pain, you might just want to blame your cingulate cortex. Of course, none of these brain areas are bad in and of themselves, nor are they solely responsible for your pain. It's just fun to point the finger at something besides your back.

So, how do these brain structures exert their influence outside your head and inside your body? After all, you're reading this because you have back pain, not head pain!

Remember when you were like ten years old and had to take that awkward class about puberty? Remember the pituitary gland? The pituitary gland is a tiny structure located right in the center of your head, yet it releases two hormones that kick off virtually every change in your body as you transition from a kid to a teenager with bigger muscles, bigger pimples, and way bigger dating problems.

When the brain interprets threats as pain, and especially when a significant amount of fear is involved, it will release a cascade of hormones that can drastically affect what you feel and how your body is physically behaving. Typically, it looks something like this: The brain interprets a situation as threatening. Combined with a few traumatic memories of similar threats, the amygdala and hypothalamus communicate with the pituitary gland to release adrenocorticotropic hormone (ACTH) into the bloodstream. Soon thereafter, the adrenal glands get a hit of ACTH and are spurred to release the stress hormones cortisol and adrenaline.

Normally, these hormones work in the short term to help your body make physical changes that allow you to do things like fight off attacking lions, which we know many of our readers have had to deal with. More often, they help us rocket through our morning routine when we wake up late and still need to get to work on time. They do things like direct blood flow to our skeletal muscles while taking blood flow away from our gut.

But what happens when the impetus is not something that quickly comes and goes? What if the threat that starts the cascade is something as commonplace and repetitive as bending your back to do housework or sitting in an office chair? That quick-response cortisol system gets fatigued and ends up making it much more difficult to heal (cortisol is a critical hormone in the healing process). This often creates a vicious cycle that worsens over time. Just think about it. The threat makes you temporarily less able to heal. Because you don't heal, the tissues that feel threatened continue to stimulate the brain for fight or flight. And so on and so on.[6]

Another way the brain can prolong and promote pain is by stimulating inappropriate inflammatory responses within tissues. As we discussed earlier, inflammation and its related experience of increased sensation, increased swelling, redness, and warmth all contribute to our remarkable ability to heal. But what if the tissue isn't actually damaged? What if healing has already occured? This type of inflammatory response would be like if you had just demolished an old building, rebuilt your dream vacation home on top of it, and the very next day discovered that another wrecking crew had been mistakenly summoned to destroy your brand-new home. This occurs because the communication between the peripheral nervous system and central nervous system has decayed to the point where the brain can no longer

---

6   "Chronic stress, cortisol dysfunction, and pain: a ... - PubMed." https://pubmed.ncbi.nlm.nih.gov/25035267/. Accessed 20 Aug. 2020.

Chapter 3: Turning Pain Science Into Plain Science

accurately assess when tissue is damaged and when it is healthy.

At this point you may be a little overwhelmed. You may feel like your brain and body are so far gone in this terrible cycle that there is no coming back. In fact, you may be feeling more danger than before you started reading this chapter. But think back to Safety Steve and Danger Dan. Think back to Cool Hound Luke's and Murphy's Lawn Care Emporium.

When you have a problem of dysfunctional danger in the brain, the best way to treat it is with extravagantly safe experiences and thoughts. Here are a couple of safe thoughts now:

1. My back is probably not nearly as damaged as it feels like it is.
2. My dangerous and fearful thoughts about what I feel can be met with learning new information (just like everything I've read in this chapter).
3. There are a number of established behaviors that can help my body feel safe again, reduce dysfunctional inflammation, and even heal that which is still broken. All I need to do is keep reading to learn how.

The next chapter is full of safety-promoting thoughts and explanations connected to specific structures in your body and diagnoses you may have previously thought scary.

So here's to a new, safer, and better way of thinking.

Chapter 4: Structural Integrity

Now that you've got some solid pain science under your belt, you are way too smart to think of your pain as coming from a specific tissue like a disc, muscle, or joint. Nonetheless, we are going to touch on how specific tissues like these get damaged and heal. Why? Two reasons. First, we want you to understand the amazing healing ability and durability of your body. You are a healing machine! Second, we know some people will skip directly to this section to better understand the area they think they have injured.

If you read these straight through, you should find them a bit redundant. Feel free to skim if your eyes start to gloss over.

Let's start with what is potentially the scariest and most threatening structure in the human body: our discs.

What Are Discs?

Walk into a doctor's office and you're likely to see the spine with a quarter cut out of the side. You'll see what is supposed to be the "disc" oozing out. Thankfully, this is a very inaccurate representation of what a disc actually behaves like.

Discs get all sorts of bad adjectives attached to them, like degenerative, ruptured, bulging, and herniated. These words combined with the image of a jelly donut are enough to activate the amygdala that we spoke of in the previous chapter.

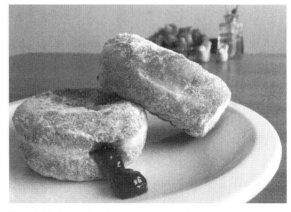

To quote a favorite book of ours, Explain Pain: "We suggest they [discs] should be called 'living adaptable force transducers' (LAFTs)... LAFTs are firmly integrated with adjacent vertebrae and are made of the same material as your ear plus some super strong ligament, just like the ligaments in your ankle."[7]

Our LAFTs are very often blamed for back pain, and it's no laughing matter! Even in PT school, we learned to think about LAFTs in isolation and were taught specific techniques to "squeeze" them back into place.

Have you ever been driving next to a big semi-truck on the freeway and happened to notice its suspension?[8]

That is some serious hardware! Sure, like anything else in this world, it can degrade over time and sometimes fail, but with proper care and maintenance, the suspension will perform well for the long haul. When we think of the serious hardware in our spines like flimsy pastry fillings, we do our design a massive disservice. If every time a trucker noticed a rusty spot on the undercarriage of their truck they junked the whole thing and quit driving, not only would we not get our Amazon Prime deliveries in two days or less, but Jimmy Hoffa would roll over in his grave (that is, unless he's still alive somewhere!).

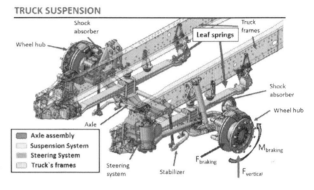

Just so you can appreciate how durable and well designed our discs are, here is a picture showing their major components and how they manage the incredible forces we put them through with ease.

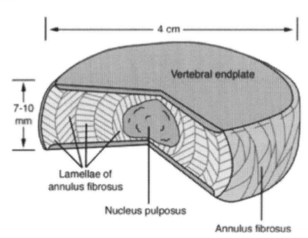

---

[7] "Explain Pain Second Edition - NOI Group." https://www.noigroup.com/product/explain-pain-second-edition/. Accessed 17 Oct. 2020.

[8] "Truck Suspension types | Car Construction - CAR ANATOMY." https://www.newkidscar.com/vehicle-construction/truck-anatomy/truck-suspension-types/. Accessed 20 Aug. 2020.

Chapter 4: Structural Integrity

As you can see, these dynamic engineering miracles have several different fiber alignments and densities, each matched to a specific direction and magnitude of force needing to be managed. In other words, whether you are bending, twisting, extending, jumping, walking, lifting, sprinting, or sleeping, there is a fiber direction for that. Pretty amazing!

So, why do discs get such a bad rap? Think back to that serious hardware underneath a semi-truck. It is appropriately designed for long miles on paved freeways with lots of little bumps and occasional big bumps. If that semi started doing most of its driving off road, causing constant turbulent bumps, it would wear out prematurely or fail. Or perhaps that truck did all of its driving on salty, wet winter roads. Oxidative processes would be accelerated and it would rust. Similarly, while our discs are more than capable of handling twisting forces, a lop-sided movement diet with constant twisting in only one direction can prematurely wear out that part of the disc. We see this often with grocery store checkers and old-school police and military folks who have been doing several hundred repetitions of Russian twist ab exercises every day for the past 40 years (seriously, these guys and gals go hard!).

When we understand the design of a disc and move congruently with that design, a disc is a durable, dependable, and undeniably awesome piece of tissue. When we don't understand, it becomes scary and a source of heightened pain. So stop confusing your spinal discs with jelly donuts. They don't live in the same universe of comparison.

What Are Bones and Joints?

Better than calling a joint a joint is to call it a joint complex. Why? Because it's complex! When we think of joints, we tend to imagine only the two surfaces that touch. For example, imagine your shoulder joint. Probably you are picturing some sort of bony white ball touching some sort of smooth concave cup. Or a knee… perhaps you are picturing a hinge from the hardware store, but made out of bones. In either case, you are not wrong, but you are missing 50% of the picture. So, as Dr. Matt used to console himself after difficult ortho exams in our PT school years, "You got 50% of the questions 100% correct." But what is the other 50%? That's the "complex" part. It is all of the connective tissue, muscles, fluids, nerves, blood vessels, and even other joints that surround and closely relate to the joint. This matters because the level at which we understand our bodies is frequently the level to which we can make emotionally connected decisions regarding their care. If all we understand about a joint is two smooth surfaces and our doctor told us those two surfaces are no longer smooth, then we are going to emotionally connect with that image and buy into a surgery that will smooth them out again. It is much better to understand that joint health is the sum of all pieces of the complex, not just those two touching surfaces.

The articulating surfaces of two bones are covered with articular cartilage, a special type of connective tissue that allows gliding, lubricated movement as well as impact cushioning. This cartilage is comprised mostly of collagen.[9] It is very possible to be missing cartilage, even

---

9   "The Basic Science of Articular Cartilage …." https://www.ncbi.nlm.nih.gov/pmc/articles/PMC3445147/. Accessed 20 Aug. 2020.

"bone-on-bone," and experience no symptoms. Actually, bone-on-bone is one of our least favorite terms because of how terrible and final it sounds.

The reason you can live a pain-free life even without cartilage is because of all the redundant stability mechanisms built into your joint complexes, like your connective tissue and muscles. Rejoice in redundancy.

What Are Nerves?

We're about to get on your nerves. These amazing structures are half ligament (for strength) and half neuron (for communication). Like the roads of a bustling metropolitan city, you have over 45 miles of nerve tissue spread out across your body. These nerves are in constant communication to and from the brain about what's going on in the body. Shockingly, all of this communication is done via electricity. Your brain sends information OUT, which produces the movements in your eyes to read this book. Your eyes send the information they are processing back to the brain so you can comprehend it.

Nerves are highly sensitive to the state of our nervous system, much like a child is sensitive to the state of their parent's marriage. If a child is in a home with a tenuous marriage, they will be more likely to become angry, depressed, and struggle with anxiety. If a child is in a home where the parents have a healthy marriage, they will be more likely to be emotionally healthy. It's the same with our nerves. If your body is in a state of stress from poor nutrition, a lack of movement, or finding out "Brooklyn Nine-Nine" isn't coming back, you'll be more likely to communicate a message of danger to your brain.

Nerves love space, movement, and blood flow. They detest stagnation, pressure, and restricted blood flow. Think of the feeling you get in your hand and arm after laying on your shoulder in an awkward position for too long. The pins-and-needles feeling comes from electrical firing in your nerves.

If you think your pain is derived from a nerve, there's no need to be nervous. Nerves are quite good at healing once you place them in the right environment. To learn more about that environment, read on to the Plan and Principles sections ahead.

What Are Muscles?

Muscles are the amazing contractile structures within our bodies that enable movement. But you already knew that. Although serious injury is rare and difficult, muscles are usually relatively quick to heal due to their excellent blood supply.

Muscles often get the blame for pain. When folks think of their "tight lower back," they are usually thinking about back muscles. They are close to the surface, and we feel as if we can "touch" them. Even though you are smart enough now to know that muscles in and of themselves are not responsible for pain, you may have experienced relief from pain when you stretched or foam-rolled a muscle. This is because tight and or weak muscles can put our body in a position that makes us more sensitive to pain, and stretching produces a feel-good reflex within our bodies. Muscles also have the incredible power to pull our body into a position of alignment and balance or out of alignment and balance. As we will see in later chapters, utilizing breath in combination with muscle activation is a powerful way to calm the nervous system and take control of your pain. Learning how to talk to our muscles is a great way to indirectly talk to our brains and coax them out of danger.

What Is Skin?

The skin is our largest organ and it's all on the outside of our body! The average person has 20 pounds of skin. The skin serves the role of gatekeeper with our environment. It's a protective barrier from the environment and an entry point for the environment. For example, our skin is a protective barrier from the carnage often involved in changing the diaper of a wiggly toddler and the main way we soak up vitamin D from the sun. Without our skin, feces or other potentially harmful bacteria could spell sickness and disease. Without our skin, vitamin D from the sun would not be turned into vitamin D internally. Research has shown increases in certain cancers, depressions, and osteoporosis when we get minimal sun exposure. Yes, that's right: Less sun can mean a higher risk for cancer.[10]

The skin is like a window into our nervous system. Have you ever had the flu and "everything hurts"? Gentle contact to our skin can be extremely uncomfortable when the nervous system is sensitized. This is a great example of the nervous system being "revved up" in response to something internal and creating an external expression through extra-sensitive skin.

The skin is rarely the culprit behind chronic low back pain. If you get a cut or other insult to the skin, it generally heals rapidly and forms a scar. Except for cases like extreme burns, the pain from skin lesions subsides quickly. Yet, in someone with low back pain, who has alarm bells blaring, the skin can become so sensitive that light touch or even air on the lower back can be excruciating. Even if the skin itself is not damaged, it can be painful. If the brain senses a strong danger threat in the lower back, it can send information down to sensitize the skin.

Our skin has many of the "danger sensors" we mentioned earlier, like chemical sensors, pressure sensors, and temperature sensors. These all play an integral role in alerting your brain to potential threats in your environment.

---

10 "Vitamin D and your health: Breaking old rules, raising new …." 17 May. 2019, https://www.health.harvard.edu/staying-healthy/vitamin-d-and-your-health-breaking-old-rules-raising-new-hopes. Accessed 20 Jan. 2020.

Chapter 5: Dubious Diagnoses

Very rarely does a patient walk into our clinic with the simple thought of "I have low back pain." Sometimes they've already talked to their primary care physician. More often, they've just had a series of sporadic consults with the renowned Dr. Google or his close affiliate, WebMD.

It's human nature to want to know WHAT is going on inside us and to attach a name to it. Sometimes these diagnoses can be helpful and reassuring, and sometimes they can increase our sense of danger and make us worse. For example, finding out that you have a simple muscle strain that will take a few weeks to heal may actually decrease the threat you associate with the injury and lessen your pain. However, finding out your back pain is related to degenerative disc disease seems like a dangerous life sentence of endless misery.

Before we deep dive into common diagnoses, it's important to remember three things:

1. Pain is about DANGER and not DAMAGE.
2. Pain doesn't come from one specific tissue like a muscle, disc, or nerve. It's always a complex interplay between our sensors, nerves, amygdala, and other brain areas. Re-read Chapter 3 if this is still confusing.
3. The best solution to solving both our danger and our damage problems comes from creating an environment of health through food, movement, and lifestyle. More on this in the coming chapters.

So, if pain rarely connects perfectly with any specific diagnosis, why did we write this section?

The information related to each diagnosis is essentially what we would tell nine out of ten clients about what they've heard they have. And the tenth? Well, there are always unique cases, but odds are you are one of the nine! We hope to bring some relative calm and sanity to terms that have been misconstrued to seem scarier and more dangerous than is necessary.

Feel free to skim this section if you don't have these specific diagnoses fixed squarely in your amygdala.

What Is Sciatica?

"I think it's my psychiatry area," Bill stated plainly, pointing towards his right butt cheek. "It always comes on when I drive." No matter what people call it, everyone agrees on one thing: It is a real pain in the behind. Sciatica is named for the sciatic nerve. Traced back to its Latin root, sciatic literally means "pertaining to the hip." So, if you have trouble pronouncing it, saying "hip nerve" is literally just as accurate. But you're not reading this section for etymology — you're reading it because you've got hip and back pain! So let's talk about that.

The sciatic nerve is the longest, thickest nerve in the body. Seriously, we've dissected these things, and they are thicker than a thumb and feel like you could use them instead of steel cables to hang a suspension bridge (please don't try this at home). The sciatic nerve starts at the spine, just above your tailbone. Its spinal roots come from L4 all the way down to S3, meaning some of its roots are in the lumbar spine and some on the sacrum (tailbone). These roots join together and make their way by the hip, through the gluteal muscles, and down the back of the thigh. Eventually it splits into two more nerves that run down the calf and finally terminate in your foot (which is a good thing, because if they didn't terminate there, we suppose you would have nerves coming out your toenails, and that sounds quite painful). Its function is to communicate sensation and movement throughout much of your leg and foot.

Like any other tissue in the body, the sciatic nerve can become irritated by excessive compression, tension, pressure, or excessive inflammatory chemicals. Let's compare it to a more familiar body part... say, a thumb. Grab one of your thumbs with the other hand and twist it until you feel tension at its base. Imagine holding this tension for days on end. Now start to repeatedly tug on the thumb and then let it go. Again, imagine this over days and weeks. Now put your thumb on a table and squish it with your other hand. Imagine if you held this pressure for as many hours a day as you sit on your butt. Are you getting the idea? Just like a thumb, the sciatic nerve is a formidable body part, but abusing it leads to pain.

Because it is a nerve, that pain can be felt anywhere along its length. This is why one of the hallmarks of sciatic is radiating pain, or pain that can be felt both at the hip as well as down the leg. Typically, sciatic nerve pain begins locally in the hip and, if it worsens, radiates down the leg. For some, the pain gets worse with prolonged sitting and better with walking, but for others, it's the opposite! It depends on what type of forces are irritating the nerve, the same way there was a difference in squishing your thumb and twisting it.

When someone comes to see us and is suspicious of sciatica, we do a series of tests to determine if the pain they are experiencing in their low back, hip, thigh, or lower leg is truly originating in the sciatic nerve, or if it is coming from a nearby muscle, for instance, the hamstrings, or if it is more an issue with the spine itself. Often it is a combination of muscle, nerve, and joint pain with a common movement or immune dysfunction. As with any medical visit, there is some obligatory poking and prodding. We also test for neural tension (excessively stretched nerve tissue), hip position, muscle strength, movement patterns, and much, much more! In any case, the important thing to know about the sciatic nerve is that it is good at healing. Even if you have had "sciatica" for a long time, it is something that is usually pretty easy to take care of with the right movements and exercise.

What Is a Muscle Spasm?

Muscle spasms go by many names, such as cramps or charley horses. They are involuntary (you can't control them) contractions of muscles that are often intense and painful. Spasms, it seems, are poorly understood by the medical community.[11] However, they seem to occur more often in people with neurological conditions, pregnant women, those doing high physical activity, or, as you may have experienced, in response to the alarm system going off in your lower back. Muscle spasms usually occur in muscles that are being asked to do a job they are not meant to or ready to do. For example, the lower back muscles will spasm more frequently in a person who uses those muscles for stability instead of using their core muscles.

Have you experienced a muscle spasm before? Maybe you were lifting weights at the gym, reaching over to pick up a toddler, or just getting up from your chair — and zap! The muscles of your back clenched up and put you in the fetal position faster than you could say "uncle." Any slight movement made your back muscles cramp again and you were left wondering if you'd ever be able to get up. Sometimes the spasms can get so intense that folks wind up in the ER. Likely they will be given a muscle relaxer like Tramadol. Usually, without intervention, the spasms decrease in intensity within a few hours and are completely gone within a few days to a week.

Muscle spasms are a bit like a teenager acting out to get attention. Instead of just telling mom and dad that they want a little more quality time and some words of affirmation, they decide to skip class and smoke some pot with their friends. Although it would seem there are less painful ways to get our attention, muscle spasms do indeed get our attention. They force us to rest, cause us to move differently, and maybe even prompt us to seek help or read a book like this one.

To decrease muscle cramps or spasms, the most important thing you can do is to create an environment of safety and security in your body using the techniques that we lay out in the Plan and Principles chapters. For muscle spasms specifically, gentle stretching and certain magnesium supplements tend to be especially helpful.

What Is a Disc Bulge, Rupture, Herniation, Slip, or Protrusion?

"Them's fightin' words!" OK, so no one has ever ridden into battle crying, "DISC BULLLLLLLLGEEE!" But these tend to be some of the scariest words in the English language.

---

[11] "Muscle Cramps - StatPearls - NCBI Bookshelf." 28 Nov. 2019, https://www.ncbi.nlm.nih.gov/books/NBK499895/. Accessed 24 Jan. 2020.

And that's a problem. All of these words are basically interchangeable. While some might say that a protrusion and bulge are used to describe a lower level of injury while a rupture, slip, or herniation describe a higher level of injury, there is so much cross-usage that it's probably not worth it to use any of them on a technical level. There are certain medical professionals who have very specific criteria for when and how they use each term, but it is rare to see consistency in definition from practitioner to practitioner. What matters most are the symptoms you experience. One person may be told they have a 3mm disc bulge, another may be told they have a lateral herniation, and a third may be told they have an 8mm protrusion. However, they may all be experiencing the exact same symptoms and severity. Part of the injury involves a sprain or load failure in the annulus (outside layer) of the disc, and part of the injury comes from impingement (when a surrounding structure is pressing on it) from the disc to the adjacent nerve root. HOWEVER, it is not a hole in a donut from which jelly is now oozing out onto the nerve root. Rather, the local inflammatory response to the damaged annulus causes helpful, healing swelling, which has the unfortunate side effect of potentially pressing on the nerve root.

Have you ever had a sinus headache? If so, were you worried that your brain was being damaged? Probably not. Sinus headaches occur when swelling in the sinuses press onto surrounding tissues, causing aching in, well, the head. Inflammation from a healing disc can put pressure on nerves, but you shouldn't worry about it any more than you would worry about sinus pressure damaging your brain.

Scoliosis/Leg Length Discrepancies

Junior high is awkward. You've got kids with hormones they don't know how to control, the first school dances, and scoliosis testing. The scoliosis test looks for a back that is raised on one side compared to the other. If one side of your ribcage or lower back is elevated compared to the other side, you likely have some curvature to your spine. This curvature is called scoliosis. If the curve is significant beyond a certain point, you may have been a candidate to wear a brace (which is not cool in junior high!), get a rolly backpack (also not cool), or even to have surgery.

Because we as humans are asymmetrical, everyone will have a spine that is slightly rotated and curved. Most curves are imperceptible to the human eye. The scoliosis curve often gets blamed on backpacks, bad posture, and hormones in adolescence. But the real culprit is our breathing! We have a respiratory system that is extremely asymmetrical. Our diaphragm on the right side of our body is two to three times larger than the left, and because of its relationship to the right-sided liver, it's set up much better for exhalation and breathing. So all day long, through our breathing, we get pulled, down, back, and to the right. Thus, the pelvis and lumbar spine get rotated to the right, and the right back side of the ribcage gets pushed back. It's not important for you to remember which direction your spine rotates with breathing. What's MUCH more important is that you understand that your breathing creates an asymmetrical pull on your spine. 23,000 times per day!

Chapter 5: Dubious Diagnoses

Being asymmetrical is not inherently problematic. In fact, our asymmetry is a good thing that enables us to respond to things in our environment quickly and without thinking which side to use. In a world where people move well, eat food in a way that communicates well with their body, and get good rest, they never get "stuck" in a breathing pattern. But because of the high volume of sitting in our culture today, the inflammatory food that makes up the standard American diet, and the constantly connected technology world we live in today, we get stuck. It's kind of like water running down a hill after a big storm. Over the course of thousands of years, a rut forms. More water goes down that part of the hill because gravity pushes it there. The rut gets deeper and the cycle continues until something changes. It's the same with our breathing. If we get stuck using the same breathing pattern, it will cause a rotational pull on our spine and lead to scoliosis.

First the bad news about scoliosis: The older you are, the less likely the rotation is to change. Now the good news: Most people we encounter who are worried about scoliosis have fairly mild versions and are able to live completely normal, active lives without surgery. Those who have had sufficiently severe scoliosis to merit corrective surgeries can also live totally pain-free lives, but some of their structural changes affect the way that their bodies move. Regardless of the extent of your scoliosis, the best thing you can learn how to do is to breathe in a way that balances our asymmetries.

Want to know the fastest way to make someone think they have an imbalanced body? Just tell them they have one leg that's longer than the other. They will forever remember and tell every health practitioner about it for the rest of their life. Heck, we even know of a few spiritual gurus whose entire ministry is based on praying for legs to grow out. Just like most scoliosis is not so extreme as to require major surgery and other life-altering treatments, most leg length discrepancies do not involve bones that are truly different lengths. Instead, asymmetries in the position of the pelvis and ribcage will cause one leg to both appear and function as longer than the other. Thankfully, this is easily correctable with a little expert guidance. We will get to this correction in the Plan section of the book.

What Is a Lumbar Strain?

Remember that time you lifted weights at the gym after a long hiatus? You put in your headphones and blasted "JUMP!" by Van Halen and got a little too ambitious on the leg extension machine. On the second rep you felt a pull in your quad muscle and immediately knew you did a little too much too soon. Or maybe you went for a long hike after being inactive for a while and tried to keep up with your teenage kids. I'll bet you woke up the next morning with some sore muscles! The painful soreness is a result of the inflammation caused by tiny tears in the muscles being perceived as threatening by the brain. These are like mini muscle strains. In the days following your workout, your body goes to work repairing the injured muscles and comes back stronger.

A lumbar strain is the term used to describe an injury to the muscles in the lower back. It's just like the muscle soreness following an intense workout but possibly with more intensity and a little more time to heal. Interestingly, even though the "damage" from working your muscles with a few sets of deadlifts in the gym and the "damage" from straining a muscle while lifting your post-college-aged child's couch for the tenth time in the last two years, the pain may be different. Here's why: when you lift weights, you expect there to be muscle soreness and you expect it to go away in a few days. When you lift a couch wrong and feel something pull in your back, you certainly were not expecting it. It's the surprise and unexpectedness of the pull that heightens your danger response system and makes the damage more painful than traditional muscle soreness from exercise.

Often "lumbar strain" is a term used for any sort of discomfort in the lower back. You see, it's really tough to isolate exactly what structure in our body is producing pain. Like we mentioned before, pain is produced by our brain in response to what it perceives as a threat. Even if it's painful to contract or stretch your lower back muscles, the issue could still lie elsewhere.

What's important with any injury is to listen to your body. Take time to rest and contemplate what led to you getting injured in the first place. Then go about fixing the root cause of the problem.

What Is Chronic Injury?

Chronic injury is simply an injury that has lasted three months or more. While it may have had a specific starting point like a car accident, it often is insidious, or without a specific start point. Think back to the injuries you sustained as a little kid. Can you think of any that caused pain that lasted longer than three months? Typically, children's bodies are much better at healing than adults. Even if they have poor diets and environmental factors, their mother's bodies selflessly gave them enough raw material to carry them through the first several years of life with near magical regenerative abilities.

By the time we reach adulthood, this planet has taken its toll on us. We are often nutritionally depleted, physically and psychologically stretched thin, and stressed out. This makes it much more difficult for our bodies to fully heal after being injured. To make matters worse, we often are totally oblivious to the injuries we are sustaining! Take sitting for example. Nobody ever broke their back by sitting down, right? Wrong! Prolonged sitting places unbalanced loads on the spine and surrounding tissues that gradually suffocate them of blood flow, starve them of nutrients, and distorts their original structure. But this doesn't happen all at once, the way falling off a ladder or getting rear-ended does. In either case, the real question is: Why does the body not heal in a normal time frame? Part of the answer is in the impaired healing system, and part in the impaired daily movement and postural habits.

Now let's consider a straightforward injury like a muscle strain from doing a set of deadlifts wrong at the gym. In a normal, healthy healing system, the back muscles heal and the pain subsides in a few weeks. But in a dysfunctional healing system, the pain persists long after the original injury should have healed. This is because the nervous system is extra sensitive due to stress, poor movement, bad diet, etc.

Chapter 5: Dubious Diagnoses

But maybe you have back pain and you never sustained an injury. It just sort of started a few months, or years, ago and it's never gone away, or it's gotten worse. Pain of this sort is usually associated with accumulated minor injury and re-injury due to habitual dysfunctional movement and postural strategies. Consider this example: A 50-something man bends forward every day using only his back to tie and untie his shoes. It's never given him any trouble, until one day it starts to bug him a bit. Fast forward a few years later, and he can barely bend forward at all. The accumulation of poor movement coupled with a sedentary lifestyle and bad nutrition habits has led to his brain perceiving the bending forward movement as extremely dangerous.

What Is Chronic Pain?

Similar to chronic injury, chronic pain has a time frame of three or more months. As far as definitions go, that's about it! However, you can read on if you would like a little discussion in addition to a definition.

Chronic pain is often directly linked to chronic injury. However, we felt it merited its own section because we want to make it abundantly clear that pain and injury are two independent events. In case you have just skipped to this section and have not read Chapter 3, we like to say that pain means danger, not damage. It is a complex psychological construction that ties together memories, emotions, worldviews, and many other unique, personal factors along with actual somatic (bodily) sensory input to make its best guess at whether or not something is safe or dangerous. In other words, two people could go to the doctor to receive a vaccine, receive the exact same poke in the same spot on their shoulder, and for one it would be a tiny sting, and for the other, a traumatic stab. In the first person's mind, the situation was fundamentally safe, and the mind provided a reasonable alarm response. For the second person, the situation was fundamentally dangerous, and the mind provided a blaring emergency alarm response. Similarly, imagine a person who was mauled by a dog as a child. That traumatic memory will play a huge role in constructing the magnitude of alarm response when nipped by a tiny Chihuahua.

Because pain is essentially a psychological construction, mental health plays a huge role in the type of pain you feel, how long you feel it, and how helpful or unhelpful that pain is to your daily life. Pain that motivates helpful, protective change in action or behavior is ideal. Pain that is either insufficient to motivate necessary change, or, more commonly, excessive to the point of crippling even healthy behavior is dysfunctional and must be addressed.

Phantom limb pain is an excellent example of excessive pain. Phantom limb pain is pain felt in a limb that no longer exists, for instance, in a veteran who has had a leg amputated. Even without any tissues to be injured, without any nerves to communicate sensation, the brain still constructs a painful experience.

This is one of the reasons why so many surgeries for chronic pain are unsuccessful. Just removing a piece of damaged bodily tissue does not necessarily prevent that area from aching. Even a nerve block cannot always stop what the mind constructs. As I am writing this, I just received a message from a client with back pain who received a nerve block last week. He was letting us know that his pain is exactly the same. Tragic! But if pain can be understood and dealt with according to its nature, all hope is not lost. If you have had pain lasting longer than three months, it is time to see an expert and figure out what's going on.

What Is Fibromyalgia?

If you suspect you have fibromyalgia, or have recently received it as a diagnosis for your chronic pain symptoms, I have some extremely good news, and a little bad news.

First, the bad news… There is no magic cure, pill, surgery, exercise, or superfood for the pain you have.

Here is the extremely good news: If you want to get better, you can.

First, you must understand the nature of your pain, because it is quite different from most illnesses. Most injuries follow a pattern that any child is familiar with: First, some sort of tissue insult occurs. It could be a burn on a stove, a skinned knee, or perhaps a sprained ankle or broken bone. Second, proportionate to the severity of damage (or so it appears; more on this later), a local inflammatory response occurs, causing characteristic swelling, redness, warmth, and sensitivity. Third, the inflammatory response cools down and the damaged tissue begins to look better. Fourth, the inflammatory response goes away completely, and the tissue looks back to normal, or perhaps has some scarring. This process typically takes about 2 weeks for small injuries, 6 to 8 weeks for moderate injuries, and 12 weeks for severe injuries.

But fibromyalgia behaves differently. You may have already taken a trip (or several) to your primary care physician and been met with vague explanations and furrowed brows. Physicians educated in Western medicine hate complex pain. A very brief lesson in philosophy reveals the reason: Since the Renaissance, Western science has used the philosophical tool of reductionism to solve medical problems. Reductionism is the belief that complex problems can be divided into smaller, simpler pieces. These pieces can, in turn, be analyzed, manipulated, and understood. If you ever competed in a science fair or took a high school science course, chances are you were instructed in a reductionist philosophy. It is the backbone of the "scientific method." In medicine, reductionism looks at an illness as having a single source cause that must be identified and eliminated. This philosophy has resulted in many great breakthroughs: Polio, smallpox, and diphtheria are just a few of the killers now all but eliminated by modern vaccination.

But there is a growing pain pandemic that reductionism has failed to address. Ironically, the medical system is so utterly locked into reductionism that they have attempted to define certain chronic pain conditions, in this case, fibromyalgia. I am hinting, and will now state plainly, that fibromyalgia is not a typical diagnosis, as its diagnostic criteria are woefully lacking in specificity and prognostic value. That's why your physician is so frustrated. Even the characteristic "18 tender points" are points that will be tender on just about any human. Any human!

On the positive, giving it a recognizable name does allow for insurance to pay for treatment. But what is the treatment? Currently, treatment for chronic pain is either too vague — diet (full of misinformation), exercise, and positive social relationships (thanks, Mom!) — or too dangerous — NSAID overuse and worse, addictive opioids and their kin. There has got to be a better way!

There is. Like most things in life, if you want to find something hidden, you have to know where to look. Western medicine simply looks for solutions in the wrong places! Our Plan and Principles sections lay out the steps you need to take to solve fibromyalgia.

What Is Degenerative Disc Disease?

"Them's fightin' words!" OK, so no one has ever charged onto the battlefield yelling, "DEGENERATIVE DISC DISEASE!" But if they did, it would probably strike fear into the hearts of their enemies. Assuming their enemies were modern, middle-aged Americans. What's that? I already used this joke in the disc herniation section? Good memory. So, what is it?

Well, first of all, it is not any more a disease than gray hair or wrinkles. It's just regular aging. For those with healthy lifestyles and low stress, the years can be kinder. For those with poor lifestyles and chronic stress, the effects of aging can occur sooner. So, while it is important to do your best to take care of your body, sooner or later we all age, and part of that aging occurs in the discs. While hair gets grayer and thinner, discs get drier and smaller. This reduces their ability to manage forces between vertebrae. On a performance level, this means the spine is less able to cope with major strains, like landing from a big jump or riding a jet ski. On a preventative level, it means the spine is less able to handle insults like bad movement ergonomics (read: lifting from the back and not the hips) or car accidents.

However, normal age-related changes to the spine are not a sentence to chronic back pain. A fully bald man with white hair coming out of his nose and ears may not make the cover of GQ magazine, but that doesn't mean he can't put on a nice suit and still look rather dashing (he may need to trim that nose hair a little bit…). The bottom line is: If you have degenerative disc disease, you do not have a real disease. If you have pain, it is likely due to other, controllable factors.

What Is Spondylolisthesis?

There are numerous medical terms that start with "spondy." You've got spondylolisthesis, spondylosis, and spondylitis, just to name a few. "Spondy" comes from the Greek "spondylo," which means vertebrae. Generally, this collection of terms is used to refer to a forward push of the lumbar spine. In our experience, patients are often shown their X-ray of their lumbar spine, given a diagnosis of spondy-something, and told their vertebrae are slipping forward! Now if that's not scary, I don't know what is!

Thankfully, most — yes, most — folks with spondylolisthesis live pain-free lives. This is because their condition is not sufficiently dangerous for their brain to perceive a threat. Furthermore, even if you do have pain and have been diagnosed with spondylo-something, through the postural and lifestyle changes we will talk about in the coming chapters, you can create the type of change that your body needs to feel safe and secure so you don't live in pain.

MRIs, X-Rays, CT Scans, and Other Imaging

Oof! This is a big one. Perhaps we'll make t-shirts or start a hashtag on Twitter: YOU ARE NOT YOUR MRI. A lot of people should say this to themselves every time they look in the mirror. Imaging, like MRIs, X-rays, and CT scans, can give valuable information and find life-threatening conditions, but it rarely tells the whole story when it comes to low back pain. This is especially true with regard to disc issues. Let's zoom in on a typical story...

At some point, most folks will go through a spell of back pain. Maybe they got into a fender bender, or maybe they were just bending over to pick up the morning paper. Suddenly, it's a world of pain and stiffness. Next, it's a trip to the doctor or urgent care. A high dose of muscle relaxers and a pain prescription later, and it's off to imaging. After a week of crippling, stay-home-from-work pain, you're following up with your physician. Pointing to a blurry image that apparently represents your spine, she states grimly, "You have a bulging disc at L4-L5, and it's pressing on your nerves." Sounds scary! Next she directs your attention to a plastic model of a spine with something that looks like an oozing jelly donut between two of the bones. She gestures to the oozing jelly: "This is basically what has happened at your disc." Her face is quite emotionless, like she does this all the time. And she does! Low back pain is one of the most common reasons for a trip to urgent care.

Back at home, it's just you, your back pain, and a disc of MRI images. Something about the MRI is burning a hole in your mind. It's different than when you broke your arm in high school. That was painful, but you could see the problem, and you could watch it heal. This disc thing is different. It's mysterious. It's out of sight. It cost several thousand dollars and took a half hour just to get those weird images. The report sounded so bad. Besides the L4-L5 disc protrusion, it also said you have things like foraminal narrowing, modic changes, and osteophytes — enough to make your head spin! Worst of all, you were diagnosed with degenerative disc disease.

Yikes. Let's zoom back out. If you are like most of our patients, you probably have a few gray hairs on your head. Now, nobody likes going gray, but very few are truly distressed about seeing some signs of aging as they, well, age. Just like gray hair and wrinkles, the insides of our bodies age, and the vast majority of it is totally harmless. The trouble with an MRI or X-ray is that it compares your images with that of an unblemished young adult, making it seem much worse than it is. In fact, research has shown that many people without any back pain at all have quite scary-looking findings on their imaging. In other words, if you've been around the block a few times, it's almost guaranteed your imaging will reveal things like osteophytes, modic changes, narrowing foramina, even "degenerative disc disease."

But not to worry! You are not your MRI! You are not your X-ray! It is highly unlikely that your back pain is the direct result of what was found. Remember the "damage vs. danger" message that we hammered home earlier? Happily, it is also unlikely that surgery or significant pain medications are necessary. For most people, a thorough, hands-on assessment by a physical therapist can reveal the real-time causes of your back pain as well as the road to recovery. The sooner this occurs, the less likely you are to develop chronic or debilitating pain. The longer you wait, the combination of unchecked inflammation, fear, and medical misinformation can become a steep, uphill battle.

Read on to learn how you can get pain-free and active regardless of your imaging findings.

Is This a Medical Emergency?

Listen up. It's highly unlikely, but if you are reading this book to try to get your legs to work again after you fell 20 feet off a roof yesterday on your back, you need to put it down and get serious medical attention. The following section is a brief summary of situations that merit immediate or emergency medical care.

If you have any of the following, make an appointment with your primary care doc ASAP[12]...

---

12 "Documentation of Red Flags by Physical Therapists for ...." https://www.tandfonline.com/doi/abs/10.1179/106698107791090105. Accessed 6 Feb. 2020.

When It's Time to Get In to See Your Doc ASAP

1. Recent, rapid, unexplained weight loss (if you're following the nutrition section laid out in later chapters, your weight loss is explained):	• "Recent" means within the last month. • "Rapid" is more than normal weight loss, which is about a pound a week. • "Unexplained" means there is no typical reason for weight loss. It is the most important factor in determining if weight loss is a sign of something that needs a visit to your physician. This means there are no significant changes in diet and no significant changes in activity or behavior.
2. New onset of night sweats:	• Normal reasons for night sweats are menopause and anxious or scary dreams.
3. Pain that doesn't improve with traditional therapy:	• Every once in a while, we see a patient who does not respond to anything we do. They get care, do their exercises, improve their diet, improve their sleep, and still their symptoms persist, unchanged. If you have spent several months making healthy changes in your life and had no change in symptoms, it is a good idea to check in with your primary care physician.
4. History of cancer:	• This is the number-one predictor of future cancers. • If you have previously been diagnosed with cancer and you develop insidious low back pain, it's not a bad idea to check in with your physician.
5. Immune suppression:	• You are constantly sick with any and every bug that goes around.
6. Night pain with no logical explanation:	• Specifically, you awaken during the second half of the night due to low back pain. (If you sleep on an old, lopsided mattress and get pain at night, it's logical.)
7. History of trauma:	• Such as a recent major car accident or a fall from higher than body height.
8. Saddle anesthesia:	• This is numbness and/or tingling in the area of your body that would sit on a horse's saddle.
9. Progressive lower extremity neurological deficit:	• This means losing feeling or experiencing numbness/tingling in the legs that has progressed rapidly.

Part 2: The Plan

Chapter 6: Prognosis

Before we get fully into this chapter, let's make something plain: Muscles heal in a few days to six months. Bones heal in two to three months, while ligaments take a max of one year to heal.

Tissue		Healing Time
Muscle	Exercise Induced	0-3 Days
	Grade 1	1-4 Weeks
	Grade 2	3-12 Weeks
	Grade 3	1-6 Months
Tendon	Tendonitis	3-7 Weeks
	Tendonosis	3-6 Months
Ligament Sprain	Grade 1	2-8 Weeks
	Grade 2	2-6 Months
	Grade 3	2-12 Months
Meniscus/Labrum		3-12 Months
Fracture		6-8 Weeks

These are based on population averages. But these pieces of information do not tell us much about you on their own. As we will see, they have an intellectual satisfaction, but they hardly tell the whole story. So, let's begin where most of our patients begin, with a question:

"How long will this take to get better?"

Unfortunately, this is not a straightforward question. If we were talking about a paper cut on an otherwise perfectly healthy person, no problem. If we were talking about a broken arm bone on an otherwise perfectly healthy teen, again, no problem. But we are not. We are talking about you. And you probably have something pretty unique going on, otherwise you would not be using your precious time to read this book. So, let's try to break down this question into a few useful pieces...

"How long will this take to get better?"

"How long":

The simplest part of the question. A length of time. Measurable in days to years.

"This":

The second most complicated aspect of this question. "This" usually refers to what is felt, and what is felt is pain. As we have discussed at length, there is a difference between what is felt and what is injured. Even tissues that are physically sound may hurt, while unsound tissues may not hurt. Thus, "this" really refers to a whole person: body, mind, and spirit. An injury to a disc belonging to a strong, stress-free person who regularly eats nutrient-dense foods will heal much faster than the same disc belonging to an accountant during tax season who frequently eats fast food and misses sleep. Indeed, it will probably hurt less along the way to boot.

"Better":

The most complicated aspect of the question. "Better" is defined by you. It depends on what you want. It depends on what you are willing to do to get what you want. If your goal is to return to a lifestyle that has injured your body and irritated your mind, the length of time to get "better" will be shorter, but it won't be long before you are in pain again. If your definition of better includes a whole new you, it may take longer, but it will be well worth it.

Now that we have taken what seems like a simple question and exposed its hidden assumptions, let's talk about how healing works in general and how it can work for you.

The first and most important fact about healing is the following: You are a healing machine. If you can remember this at all times, everything will be much better. If you cannot or will not believe this simple truth, the road to recovery will be much more complicated.

The second most important fact is this: For all of modern medicine's brilliance, it is barely a candle to the blinding sun of the human immune system's innate intelligence. If you can surround yourself with medical professionals who understand and respect this, you will spend less time feeling like a broken science experiment and more time like the amazing human being you are.

Third, you must release the past and embrace the path before you. Not all that is lost is recovered, and one day we all die. Cheery, right? Dwelling on what cannot be recovered will impede what can, and more significantly will keep you from attaining what may be even greater.

Do You Believe That You Can Get Better?

Do you believe that your back pain can get better? If the pain is recent or has come and gone before, this may be an easy "yes." However, if you've lived with constant pain for years or decades, it can be tough to believe it will ever go away.

Chapter 6: Prognosis

Research shows that people who believe that they can get better are more likely to experience long-term relief from low back pain.[13]

Recently, a patient of ours came in for an initial consultation. She, like most of our patients, had low back pain. As the consultation went on, she said a few things that made it seem like she didn't think things could get better. So, I flat-out asked the question, "Do you believe this can get better?"

After a pause, she replied, "I don't think so."

I answered respectfully, "Then what brought you in for this consultation today? Why would you have come if you didn't believe there was hope?"

She took what felt like a minute and finally replied with tears welling up in her eyes, "I guess I do have some hope that you guys can help me."

If you're reading this book, it means you have not yet lost hope. Otherwise, why would you be reading it? Even if you are skeptical and have tried myriad techniques to relieve pain and failed, you're still trying.

So keep hoping like Princess Leia in Episode IV: "Help me, Obi-Wan Kenobi. You're my only hope!"

Finding Your Flight Plan

Imagine you're on a plane headed from LAX to JFK in New York. The pilot comes on at the start of the flight and says, "Hi folks. I really don't know how long this thing is going to take. Never done it before. Could be three hours. Could be eight. I'm pretty sure we have enough gas. Anyways, sit back, relax, and enjoy!"

You'd be downright scared. Rightfully so!

What would be much better would be a pilot who says, "Hi folks. We have a 4-hour-35-minute flight ahead of us. We will hit some weather about two hours in. If our estimated arrival time changes, I'll update you. Anyways, sit back, relax, and enjoy the flight!"

That is comforting.

In order for the pilot to make a prediction like this, he needs quite a bit of information. He needs to know the plane he's flying inside and out, he needs to have done the trip numerous times before, and he needs to know the weather with much more detail than the inaccurate weather app on your phone.

---

13 "Discographic, MRI and psychosocial determinants of low back ...." https://www.sciencedirect.com/science/article/abs/pii/S1529943004004863. Accessed 6 Feb. 2020.

And the same goes for you and your low back pain. If you were sitting right in front of us, telling us your story, and we were able to do an evaluation, we could give you a very accurate prediction of how long it will take to heal.

But you're reading this book and not in front of us at this moment. Healing is a complex process, and like we defined earlier, "better" is a relative term to you. So we'll do our best to help you understand some principles so you can create your own "flight plan."

1. No matter how long you've been in pain or how bad the injury is, your body can heal!
2. Tissues with good blood supply, like skin and muscle, heal faster than those with lesser blood supply, like cartilage and bones.[14]
3. The longer you've had pain, the longer it usually takes to go away.
4. There are MANY things you can do to help your body heal faster, which we will cover in depth in the following chapters.

The Healing Human Body

The injured body goes out on a mission like Rocky Balboa in Rocky 4 to come back stronger and defeat the Russians... or heal some tissues. The body starts with what's called the "inflammatory" phase. In this phase, things get warm, swollen, and often painful. Your back may get stiff and make you feel like you need to move gingerly. This is your body's way of protecting you so that healing can start. The "inflammatory soup" that your body cooks up helps to start the healing process. And this soup is the real homemade stuff. None of that canned nonsense.

The second phase of healing is called the proliferative phase. Proliferative comes from the Latin "proles," which means "offspring" or "descendants." The body literally goes about the process of creating new cells of the same type as the injured tissue. If you've strained a muscle, irritated a disk, or fractured a bone, your body has the ability to make more of them.

The final phase of healing is called the maturation phase. This is where the newly formed cells "mature" to full strength and sometimes even stronger than the previous tissue. When you fracture a bone, it will often heal stronger than the original bone. After all, the body wants to do whatever it takes to protect itself from future issues.

What to Do to Help Your Body Heal Faster

How fast you move through these three phases can be thought of like a small town with a building fire that needs to be put out. When there is only one fire, the fire department can do its job with speed and efficiency. However, if there are numerous fires to put out, the fire

---

14 "Soft Tissue Repair and Healing Review ...." http://www.electrotherapy.org/modality/soft-tissue-repair-and-healing-review. Accessed 20 Feb. 2020.

department may get spread thin across town. They would likely call in the fire department from another city. Your body, however, does not have another city to call on. If there are numerous fires for the body to put out — like a diet high in sugar and vegetable oil, stress, lack of sleep, or poor movement — it may not have the resources necessary to heal optimally. In the next few chapters, we will dive deep into what it takes to create the ideal environment for healing or how to make sure that back pain is the only fire that needs attending to.

Chapter 7: The Get Back Up Foundations Program

Before getting started, you'll definitely want to download the free resources at getbackupbook.net. With the exercises below, a picture simply doesn't do it justice. That's why we made FREE videos for you to download for every single exercise.

We spent hours creating videos of EVERY assessment and exercise plus a bunch of bonus goodies ONLY available on the website. Go get it.

A Preface to the Foundations Program

Did you download the goodies? If not, STOP reading and do it now!

If you've arrived at this point in the book having read most of what came before, kudos to you. You're in a great place to start this back pain program and have success. If you flipped straight to the plan, we would suggest going back and reading the previous chapters to give yourself a better understanding of WHY you have pain. Understanding is an essential component of the healing process.

There are a few things to keep in mind as you make your way through this program. What we've created is a simple algorithm that matches up painful movements and most comfortable positions with the most appropriate exercises. These exercises are designed to help your body adapt and remap those movements so they become pain free.

While a can of Wolfgang Puck soup is nothing like having him as a personal chef, it's still delicious, and way better than that generic tomato soup that's been in your pantry since the Reagan Administration. Similarly, this back pain program, combined with the 12 principles in the following chapters, is the next best thing to working with us in person. It is the synthesis of thousands of successful patients, now distilled and organized around your specific needs. Even to the most cynical person, we would encourage you with the evidence-based fact that ANY exercise that does not injure you will bump you in the direction of healing.[15] And these aren't just ANY exercises!

The greatest measure of success as you embark on this path is consistency. Your ability

---

[15] "A Systematic Review of the Effects of Exercise and Physical ...." 25 Apr. 2016, https://www.ncbi.nlm.nih.gov/pmc/articles/PMC4934575/. Accessed 17 Oct. 2020.

to stick with it and keep trying even when things get frustrating will determine if you are successful or not.

So here's my challenge to you: shoot me an email at DrMatt@getbackupbook.net with the following title: "I'm Taking The 28-Day Challenge!" I get a lot of emails, but when one comes in with that title, I read it and reply.

This sounds like a simple and unnecessary step, but I guarantee it will make your success much more likely. If you're serious about doing this program, you'll email me.

The process is a bit like bamboo. Bamboo grows roots that for a long time are underground and invisible to the human eye, and then one day it shoots outward. The process of change in your body may not decrease your pain right away, but rest assured, you are digging deep roots that will eventually create long-term change.

Get Back Up Foundations Program

The assessment for the back pain program contains two very simple steps:

1. The very first step in customizing this program to you is to rank the following positions from most to least comfortable.
2. Next, rank the listed movements from most to least painful.

By doing this, you will make a foolproof progression of exercises from easiest to hardest. This is a powerful strategy for healing called "graded exposure." This method is ideal for addressing both damage problems and danger problems because it teaches your body step-by-step how to make all of your movements and positions feel safe. It also strengthens many of the smaller muscle groups that get missed over with other exercises, helping each segment of your back heal.

If it's safe, take a moment to try the following positions and movements. Then write them down in rank order.

Laying on Back (Supine)

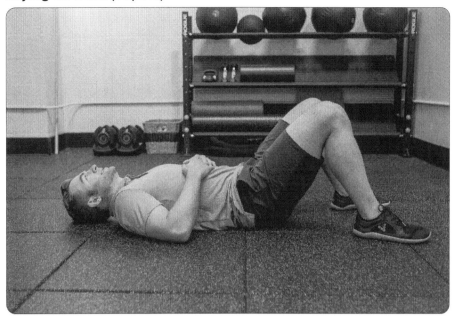

Laying on Belly (Prone)

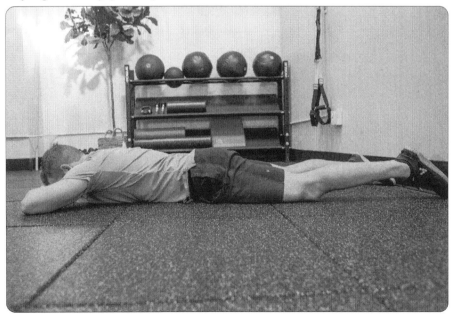

Laying on Right Side (R Sidelying)

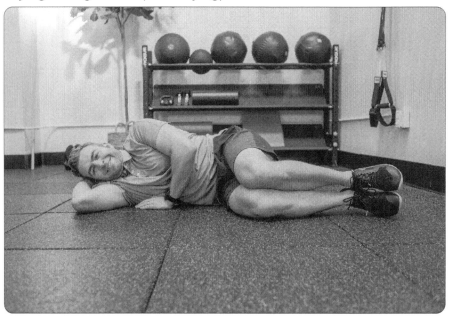

Laying on Left Side (L Sidelying)

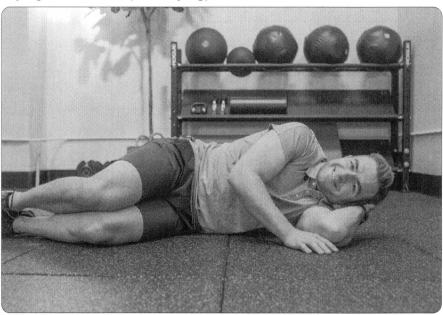

Getting on Hands and Knees (Quadruped)

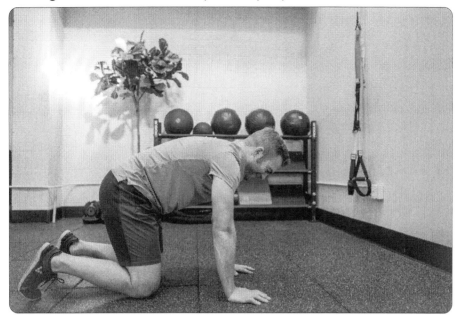

Sitting

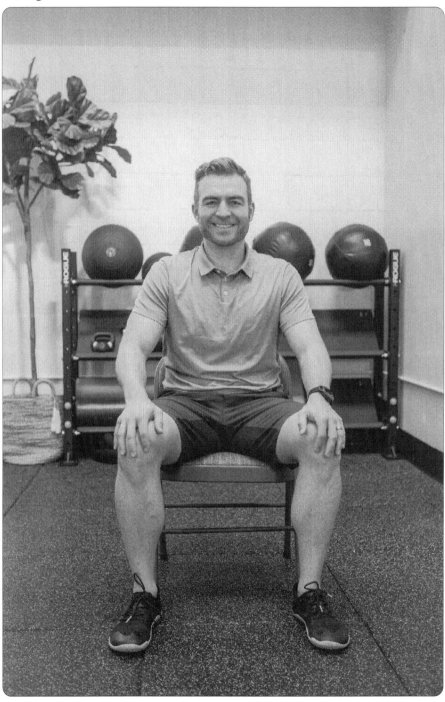

Standing

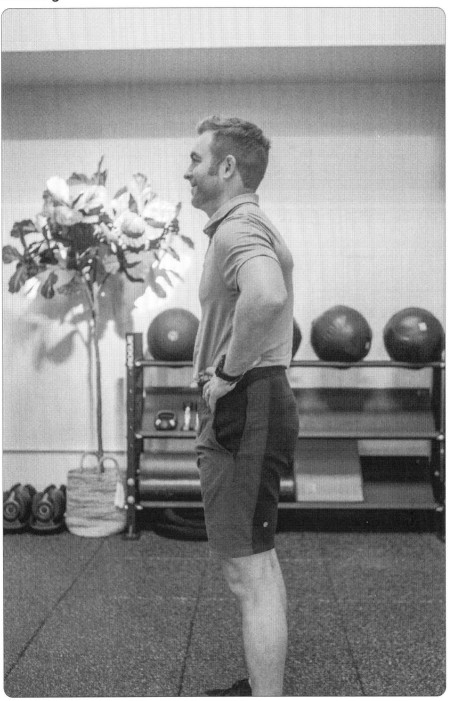

Rank movements that hurt your back:
Bending Forward (Flexion)

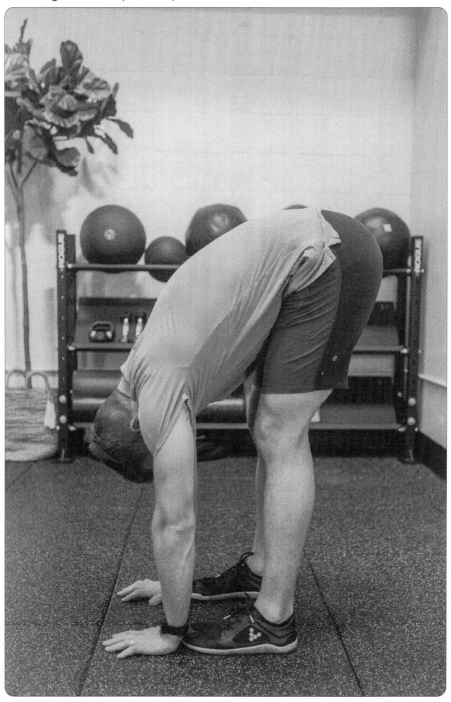

Bending Backwards (Extension)

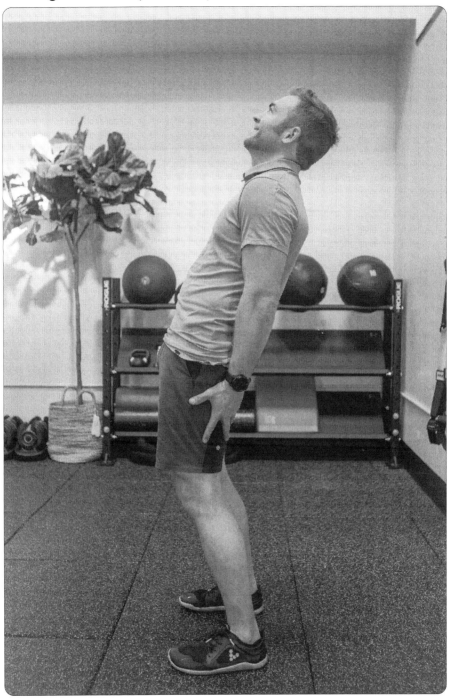

Sidebending (SB)

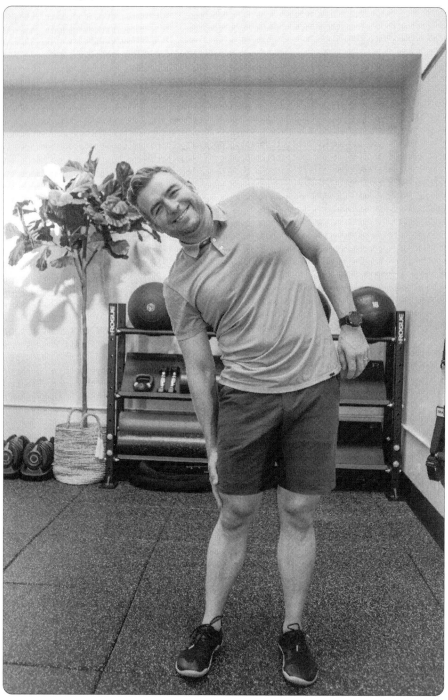

Rotating (Rot)

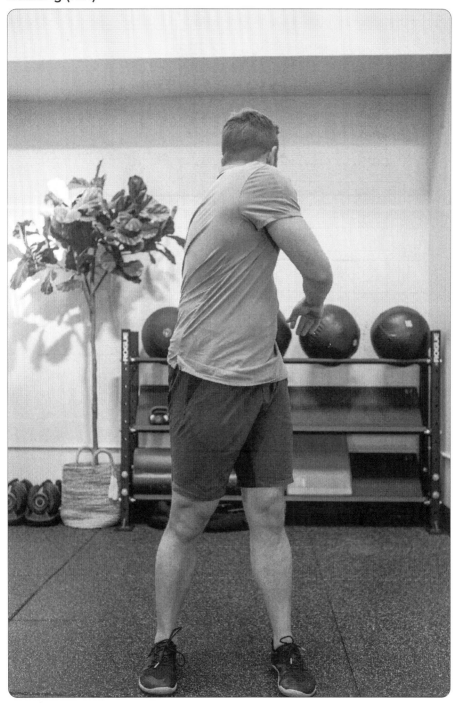

Position Rank (most comfortable to least comfortable)	Movement Rank (most comfortable to least comfortable)
1.	1.
2.	2.
3.	3.
4.	4.
5.	
6.	
7.	

If every position and movement is comfortable and pain-free, use this order:

Best Position	Supine	Prone	Sidelying left	Sidelying right	Quadruped	Sitting	Standing	
Best Movement								
Flexion	Supine Pelvic Tilt	Butt Squeezes	Knee Pull	Knee Pull	Rock Backs	Breathe and Reach	Pelvic Tilt with Exhale	
Extension free	Supine Ant Pelvic Tilt	Prone Mini Cobras	Pelvic Tilts	Pelvic Tilts	Cat Camel	Pelvic Tilt	Overhead Reach with Extension	
Sidebend	Hip Hikes	Walking Rainbows	Mermaid Rib Shift Left	Mermaid Rib Shift Right	Tail Wag	Shoulder Drops	Shoulder Drops	
Rotation	Wind shield Wipers	Baby Scorpion	90-90 Trunk Rotation	90-90 Trunk Rotation	Thoracic Rotations	Seated Rotation	Cross Body Reach	

Chapter 7: The Get Back Up Foundations Program

Videos Of Every Exercise

We decided it would be easiest if we made videos of EVERY one of these exercises. So, if you haven't already, go to getbackupbook.net to snag yours for FREE.

How to Do Each Movement:

For each exercise, set a timer for 8 minutes. Alternate between A and B until your timer goes off. Most people will go through about 4 sets of each. Going a little slower is fine. Try not to go much faster.

A. Hold and Breathe	Hold the pictured "end" position of the exercise. Continue to hold while completing 4 breath triangles.
B. Move and Flow	Smoothly move back and forth between the pictured start and end position of each exercise to complete 20 total repetitions.

How to Breathe

Simple breathing: Triangle Breathing. 4-second inhale through the nose (gentle). 4-second exhale through the mouth (forceful). 4-second pause. Repeat for 4 breaths.

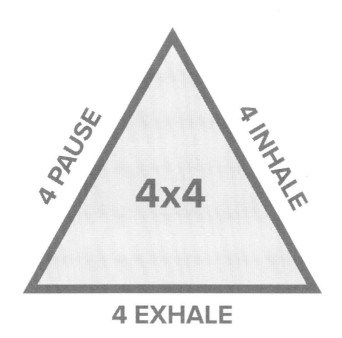

Where to Start and How to Progress

Ideally, each day, for 28 days, you'll progress from one exercise to the next, completing one 8-minute session of each of the 28 exercises in the boxes above. You'll be completing ALL the movements in your most comfortable position and then work to the next most comfortable.

What If a Movement Is Painful?

You have two options if a movement is painful. First, you can shorten the range of motion with the movement. For example, in the Supine Anterior Pelvic Tilt, you may have pain when you tilt your pelvis all the way forward, but not when you tilt 50% forward. So, start with 50% of the range. The next day, go to 50%. Spend a maximum of 5 days on a single exercise, before skipping and moving to the next one.

Alternatively, you can move back one exercise day and repeat the previous day once more before attempting the painful day again.

An Imaginary Example:

If that wasn't clear, our imaginary friend Fred will help bring clarity.

Meet Fred.

Fred has ranked his movements and positions as follows:

Position Rank (most comfortable to least comfortable)	Movement Rank (most comfortable to least comfortable)
1. Quadruped	1. Extension
2. Supine	2. Sidebend
3. Prone	3. Rotation
4. Standing	4. Flexion
5. Sidebend	
6. Sidelying Right	
7. Sidelying Left	

For Fred, his first four days will focus on movements in the quadruped position. He would start with the extension exercise in Quadruped and then do the sidebend, rotation, and finally flexion. Then, he would move to supine. Fred would perform this exercise for 8 minutes following the format we laid out above.

Starting to make sense?

Day 2 would be Quadruped Sidebend:

Day 3 would be Quadruped Rotation:
Day 4 would be Quadruped Flexion;
Day 5 would be Supine Extension;
Day 6 would be Supine Hip Hike;

So, which movement would Fred do on day 28? Yup, you knew it: Knee Pulls in Sidelying Left.

What If I Don't Have Pain with Any of the Movements?

Let's say you go through the assessment and don't have pain with any of the movements and all of the positions feel fine. Maybe your low back pain only comes on with more intense activities, like running, or more extended activities, like sitting for an hour in your car.

Listen up: You still need to go through all 28 exercises for 8 minutes a day. This is your foundation upon which everything else will build. Start here. Go through all 28 days. More often than not, you will start to notice significant improvement in your pain symptoms. As for the order, you can literally choose any you like, as long as you have spent at least 8 minutes each day doing the exercise.

Exercises

Supine

Supine Pelvic Tilt — Start:

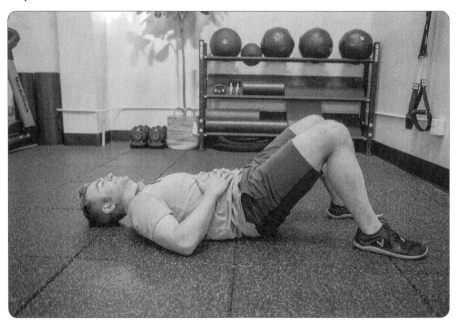

Supine Pelvic Tilt — End:

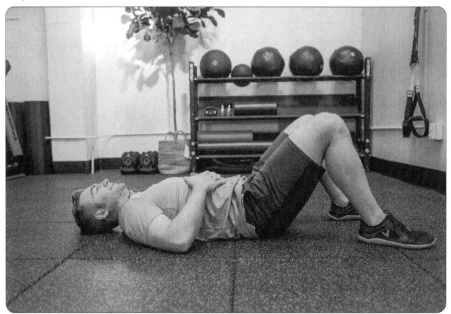

Supine Anterior Pelvic Tilt — Start:

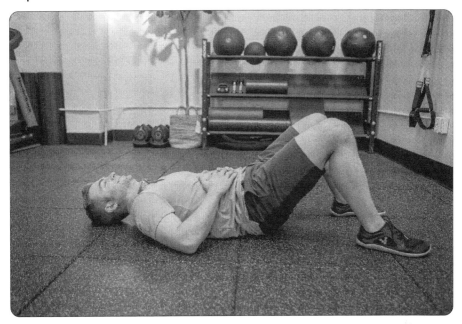

Supine Anterior Pelvic Tilt — End:

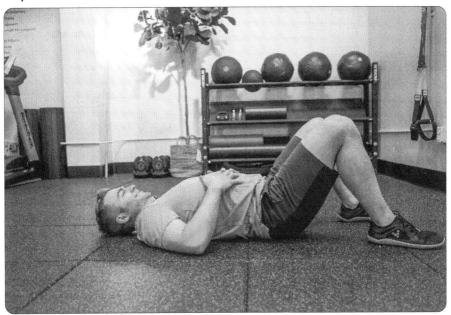

Hip Hikes — End:

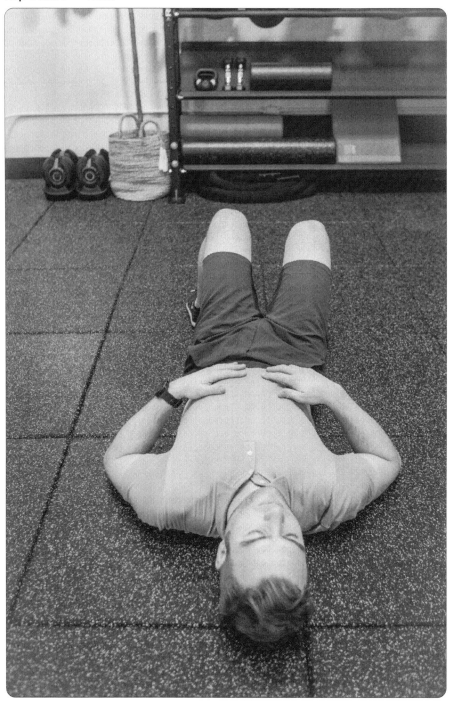

Windshield Wipers — Start:

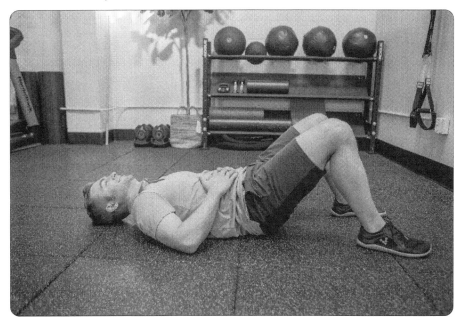

Windshield Wipers — End:

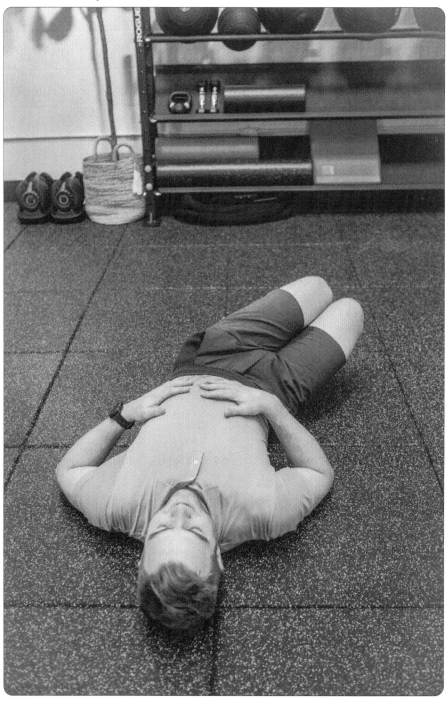

Prone

Prone Butt Squeeze — Start:

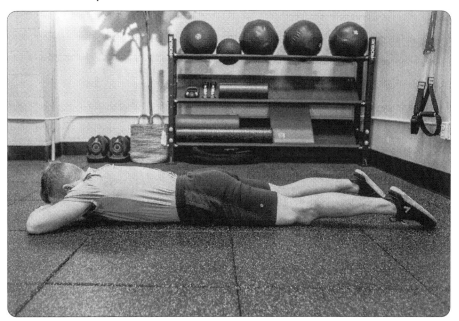

Prone Butt Squeeze — End:

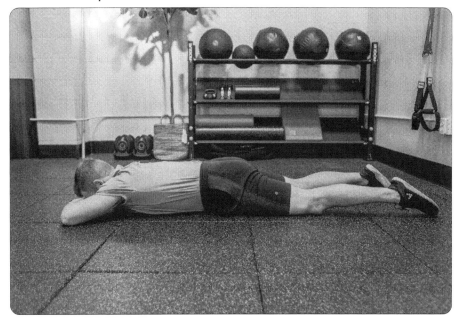

Prone Mini Cobra — Start:

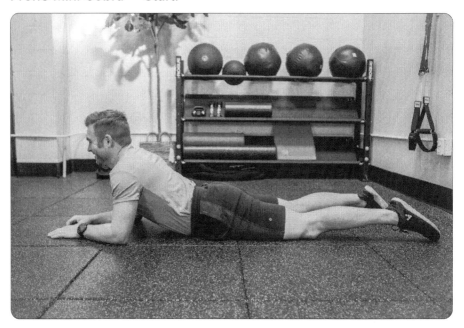

Prone Mini Cobra — End:

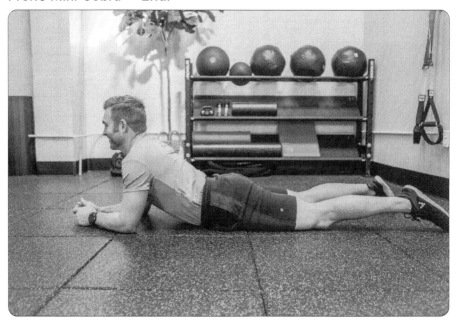

Prone Scorpion — Start:

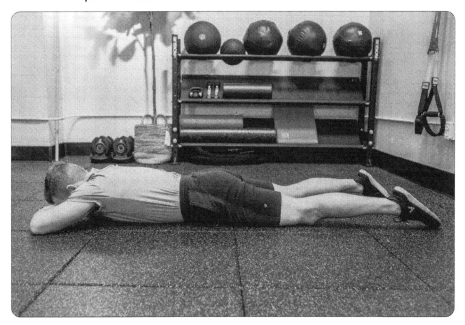

Prone Scorpion — End:

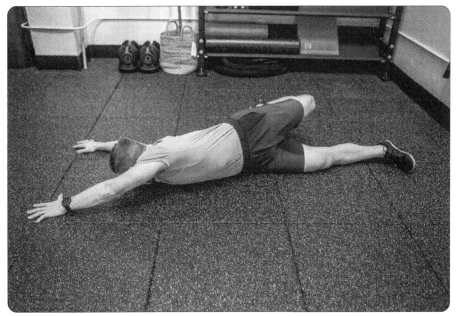

Prone Walking Rainbow — End:

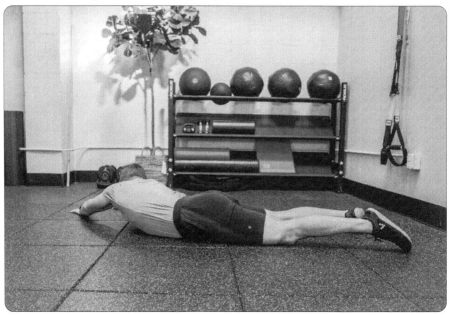

Sidelying

Sidelying Pelvic Tilt — Start:

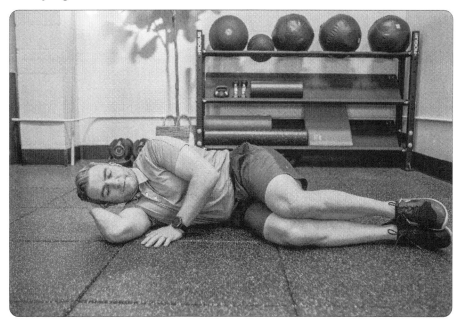

Sidelying Pelvic Tilt — End:

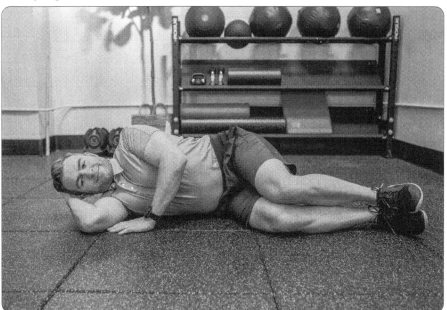

Sidelying Knee Hug — Start:

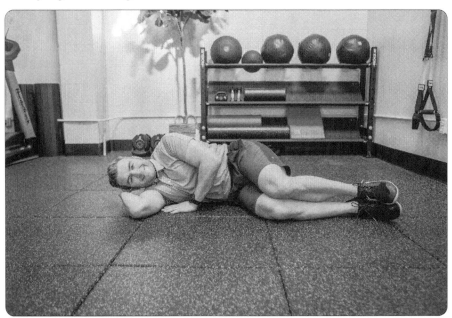

Sidelying Knee Hug — End:

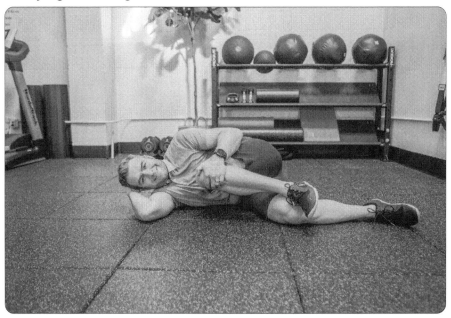

Sidelying Trunk Rotation — Start:

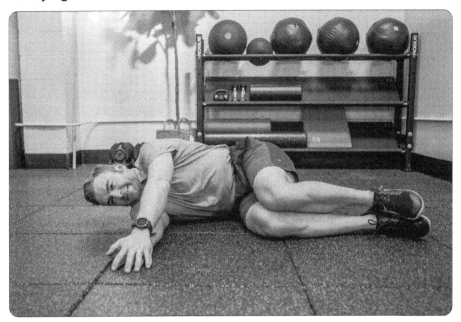

Sidelying Trunk Rotation — End:

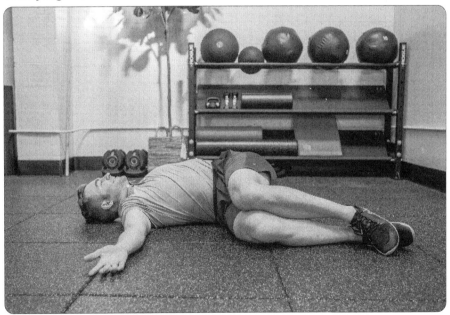

Mermaid Rib Shift — Start:

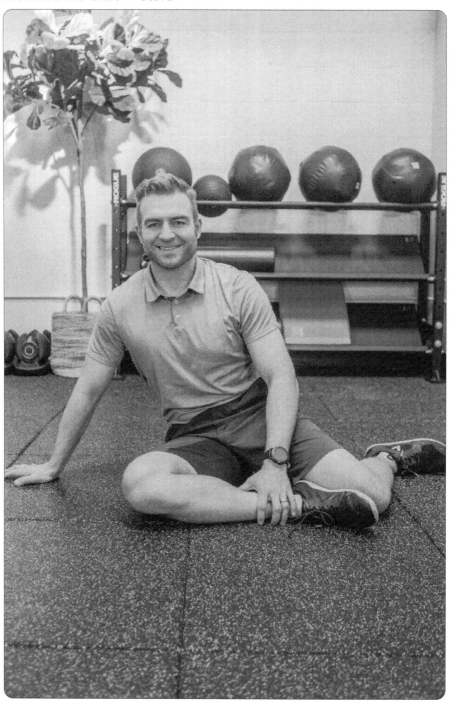

Mermaid Rib Shift — End:

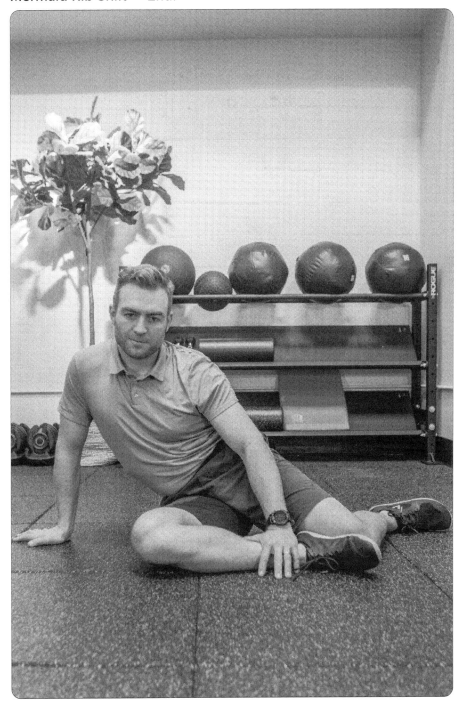

Quadruped

Quadruped Rockback — Start:

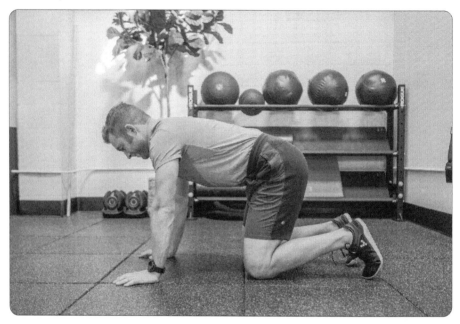

Quadruped Rockback — End:

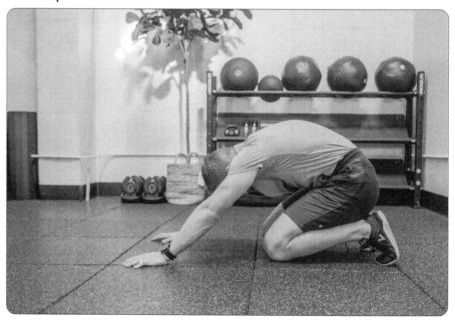

Quadruped Cat Camel — Start:

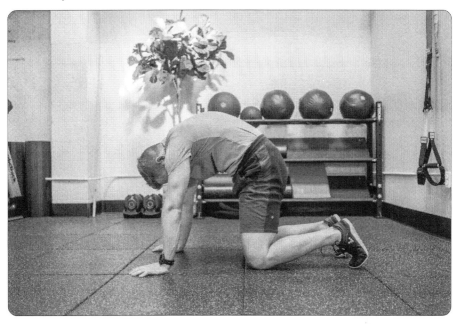

Quadruped Cat Camel — End:

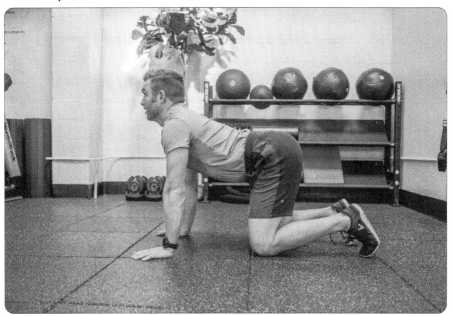

Quadruped Tail Wag — End:

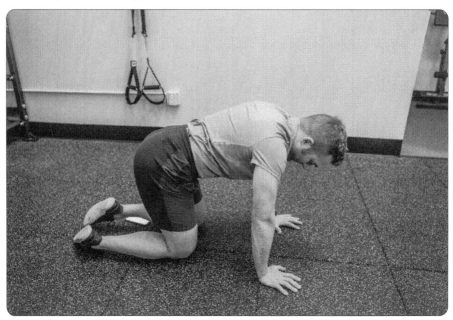

Quadruped Thoracic Rotation — Start:

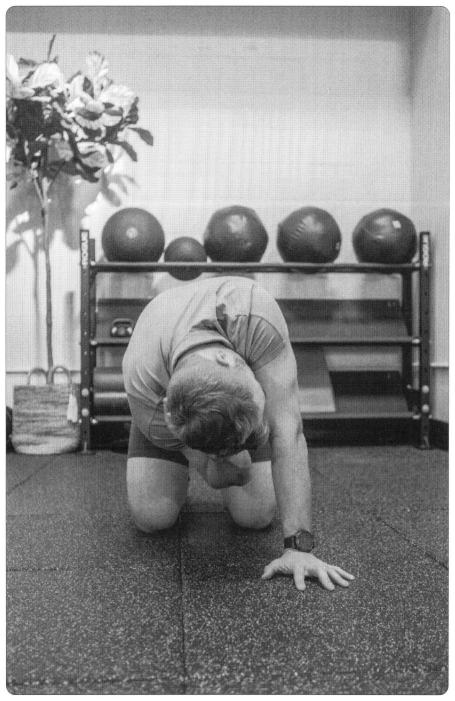

Quadruped Thoracic Rotation — End:

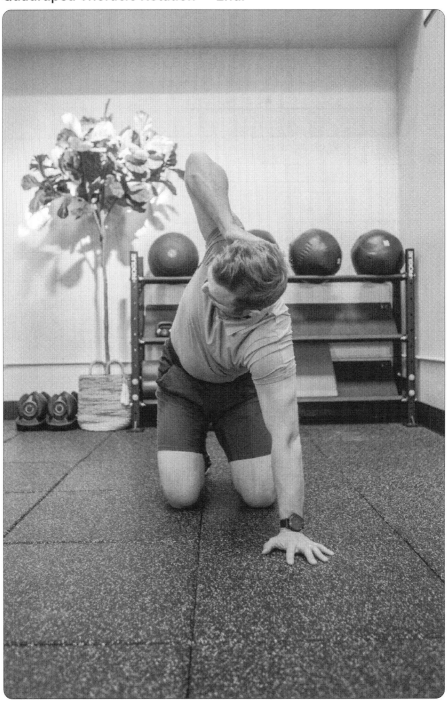

Sitting

Seated Breathe And Reach — Start:

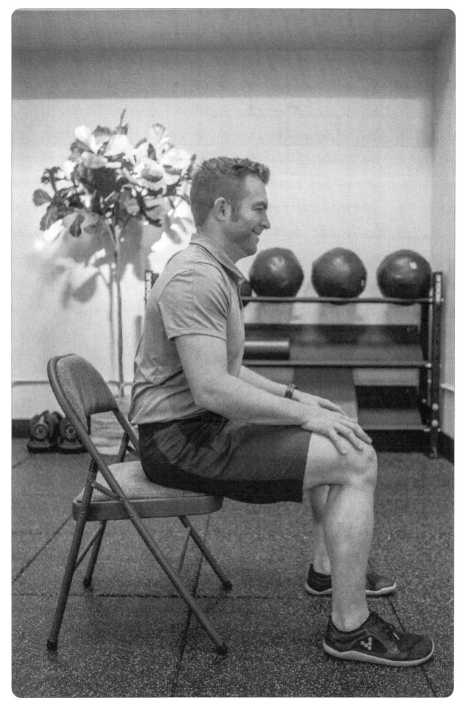

Seated Breathe And Reach — End:

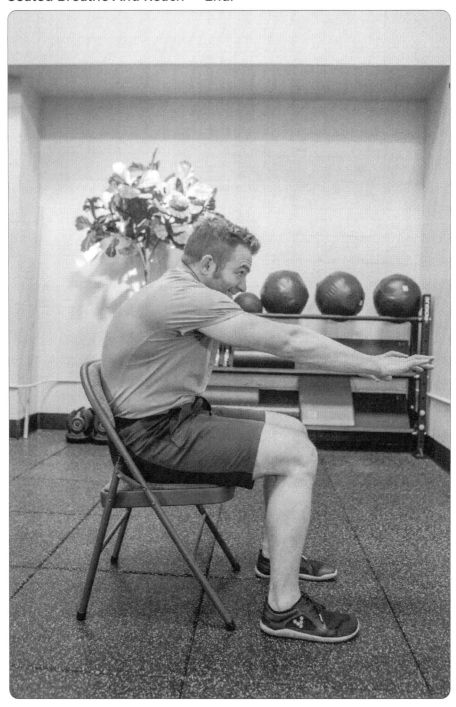

Seated Anterior Pelvic Tilt — Start:

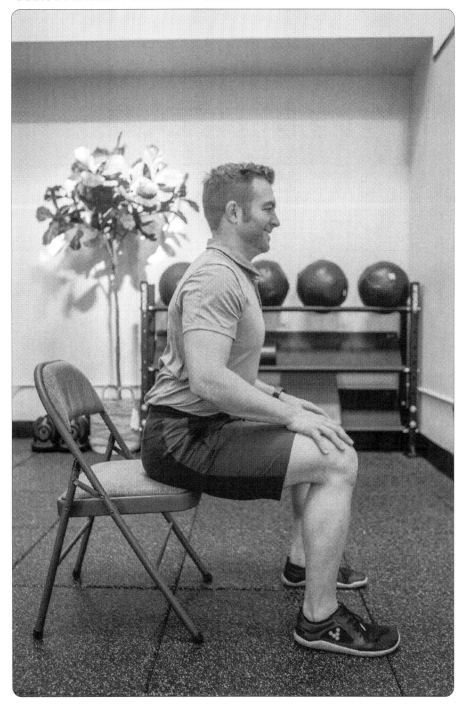

Seated Anterior Pelvic Tilt — End:

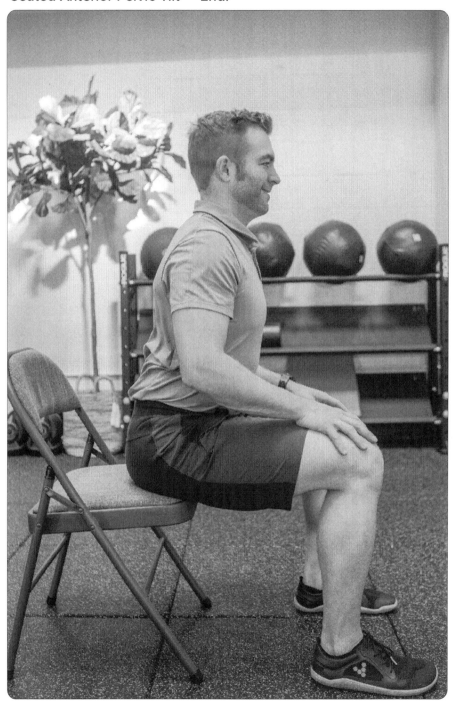

Chapter 7: The Get Back Up Foundations Program

Seated Shoulder Drops — Start:

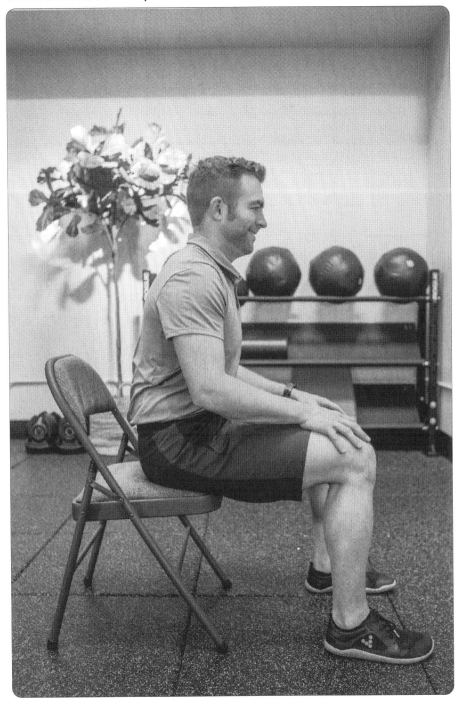

Seated Shoulder Drops — End:

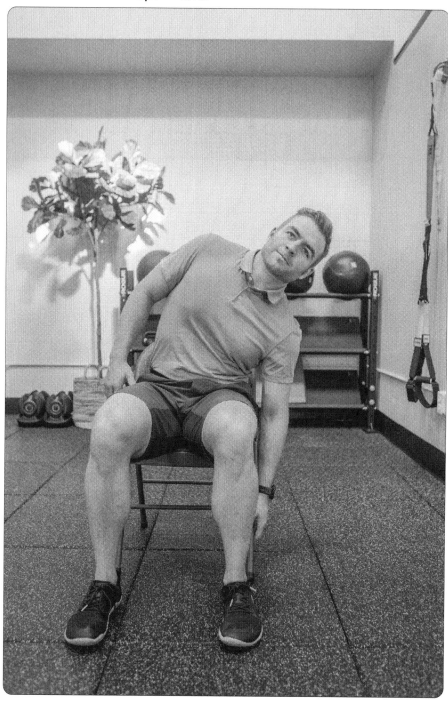

Seated Rotation — End:

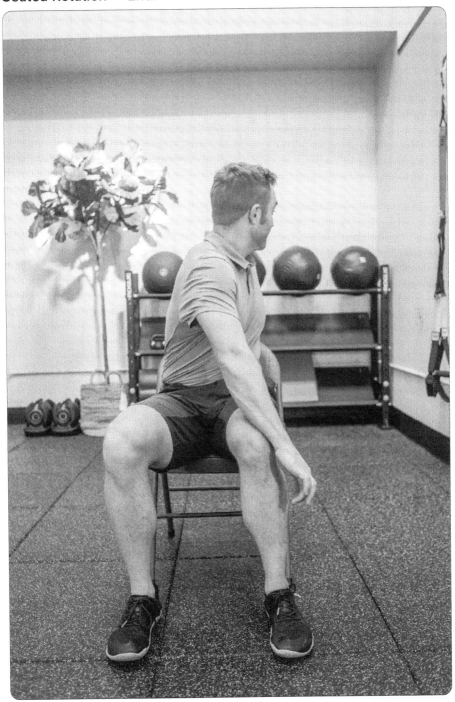

Standing

Standing Pelvic Tilts — Start:

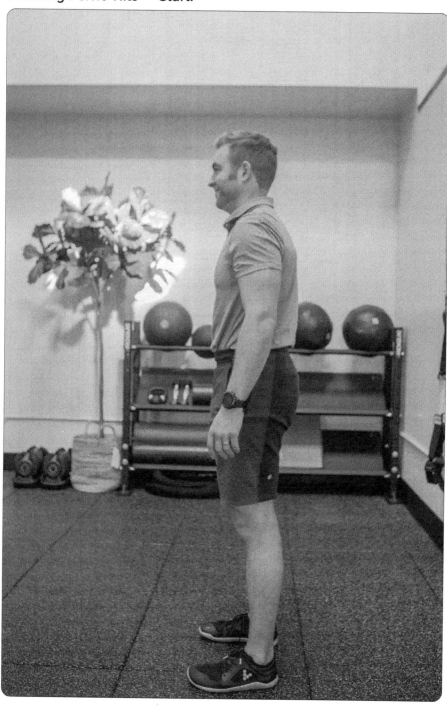

Standing Pelvic Tilts — End:

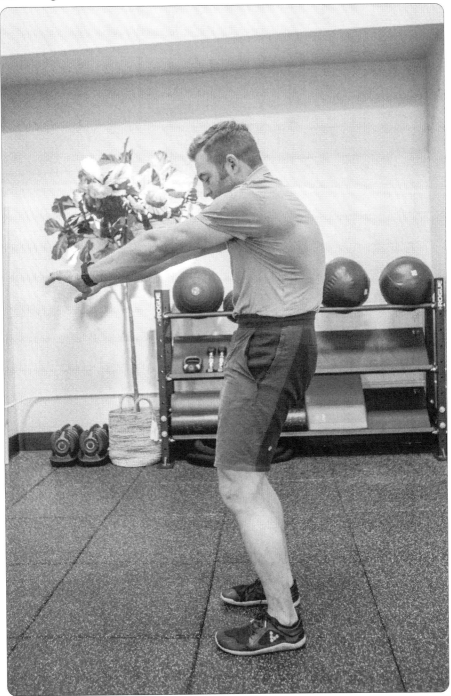

Standing Overhead Reach — Start:

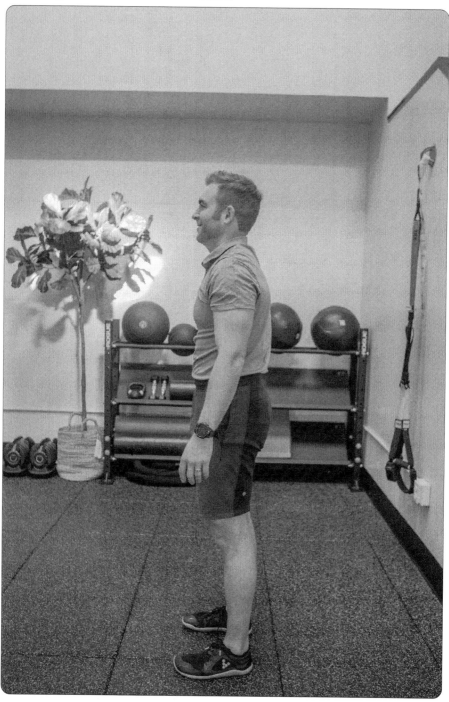

Standing Overhead Reach — End:

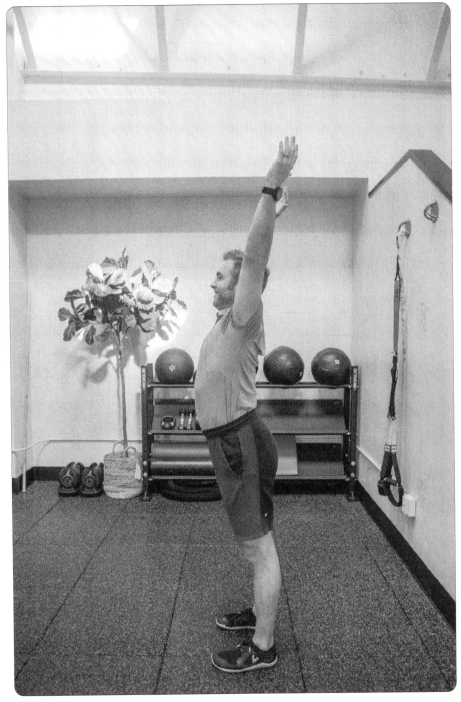

Standing Cross Body Reach — End:

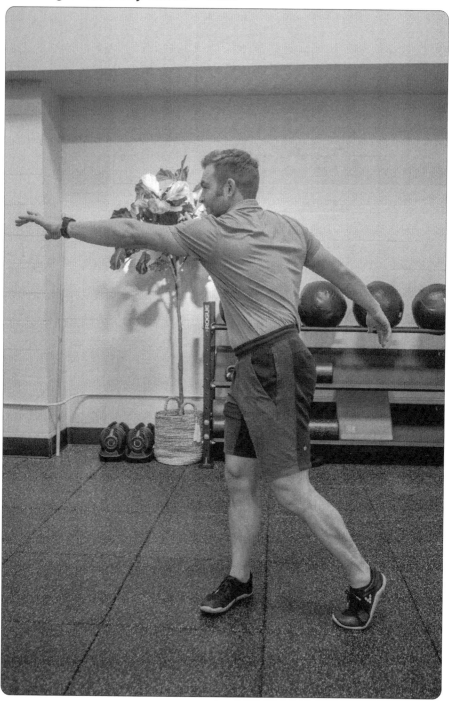

Standing Shoulder Drops— End:

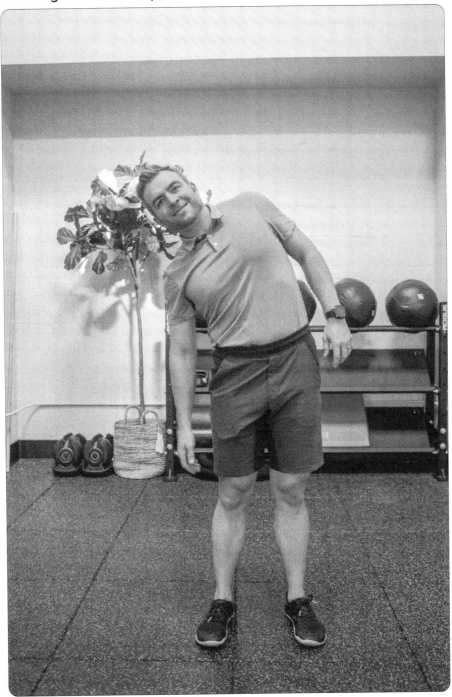

What If I Complete Phase 1 and Still Have Pain?

If you diligently complete this program for the first month and have not experienced significant improvement in your symptoms, reach out to us via email at DrMatt@getbackupbook.net.

What's Next?

Congratulations and welcome to a very exciting new chapter! If you've completed 28 days (or more!) of our Foundations Back Pain Program, it's worth some time to look back at what you've accomplished.

I have a special gift for you if you finished the program. Simply shoot me an email at DrMatt@getbackupbook.net with the title "I Finished The Foundations Program!" with your mailing address in the body of the email.

It's time to celebrate what you've accomplished! First you gained clarity on which movements feel safe and which are uncomfortable. Then you prioritized and protected 8 minutes every single day to go through a strange, new exercise. You breathed deeply, you moved gracefully (maybe), and you pelvic-tilted like it was your job. You may have garnered a few strange looks from family and a few frantic licks from your dog. But you persevered through the dog kisses and the raised eyebrows for 28 days. Now it's time to turn the page and start the next chapter.

It's time to get acquainted with the new you and set some lofty goals. It's also time to begin a training program that will help you grow in physical performance and bullet-proof yourself from future injuries. Unfortunately, finding a great training program is a bit of a needle in a haystack. But don't worry. We've got your back!

If what you've received from us so far has helped you and you're not completely sick of our jokes, and if you're feeling a little sad that this ride is coming to a close and wondering how you can keep building momentum and growing into the best version of yourself, we have good news.

We've created the most amazing, comprehensive training program called V23. It takes you on a 12-week journey of fitness, nutrition, and lifestyle coaching based on our highly successful Village model. At the writing of this book, it is the ONLY comprehensive training program written by doctors of physical therapy. The best part is that you can try it now absolutely free for two weeks.

Just enter in the link below and get ready to learn how far your body can take you and how good you can feel getting there!

Villagefpt.com/V-23-Trial

Chapter 8: Balls, Core, And Stretches Galore

Please, we beg, go to getbackupbook.net and download the FREE resources associated with the book. They contain a video explaining EVERY one of these mobilizations, stretches, and core exercises below.

In this chapter, we lay out the best mobility exercises, stretches, and core routine for beating back pain. If you've done the Foundations Program in the previous chapter, these exercises are an awesome next step.

But first, let's answer an important question: Should you do mobility exercises and stretches?

Definitely.

Here's a tip though: Don't make your objective with these types of activities to increase your mobility.

Wait, what? Do mobility exercises but not to increase mobility?!

Generally speaking, these exercises are great and often helpful for relieving pain symptoms. However, mobility is not straightforward. For example, many of our clients come in complaining that their hamstrings are tight and stiff. Many of them have been doing exercises to get more flexible, mobile, or looser hamstrings. However, when we actually assess them, it turns out their hamstrings are already way too long. The tightness they feel is actually coming from the position of their pelvis, which is pulling the muscle apart from its other attachments below the knee. Ironically, the cure for their tight hamstrings is actually to shorten and strengthen them, not increase their mobility!

Another important example of why mobility is not a straightforward concept is found at the spine itself. Often a segment that is stiff is immediately neighbored by a segment that is too mobile. Rather than the stiff segment, it is the mobile segment that gets extra wear and tear, causing irritation and pain, and eventually instigating an inflammatory response that makes the whole bodily region ache and feel... stiff!

The bottom line is that the body's need for mobility and stability can be tricky to understand.

On your own, it's better to make your objective to stimulate your muscles and joints and let your body's intelligence take care of what moves and what doesn't.

Let's put that into context and bring back the hamstring situation.

Do:

1. Foam Roll the hamstrings with moderate intensity.
2. Pair a mild hamstring stretch with a mild hamstring activation (e.g. gentle supine hamstring heel to ceiling, followed by heel dig or glute bridge).

Don't:

1. Use a foam roller or similar to beat your hamstrings into submission.*
2. Stretch your leg as far as it will go, hold it there as long as possible, and/or bob up and down like an old-school track athlete.

*We have a client whose catchphrase for any spot on her body that is bothering her is "I want to kill it." And she applies this desire liberally to her foam rolling if we don't gently persuade her to be kind to her body.

The reason the "Do" works is because it allows the body's soft tissues, joints, and related nerves and blood vessels to be stimulated without being threatened or permanently deformed. In turn, the body's innate healing system wakes up and starts to take care of the areas being stimulated.

The reason the "Don't" fails is partly because it puts you at risk for injury, but more importantly because it prevents your body's innate healing system from working properly. It would be like a five-year-old with a big idea of how to build a rocket ship out of cardboard and bubblegum walking up to a NASA engineer and saying, "No thanks, mister, I think I can handle this."

Using Mobility Tools To Beat Back Pain

A simple tool like a mobility ball (lacrosse ball) or a foam roller can provide a positive, safe input to your nervous system and help decrease pain in the body. Below, we walk through a full-body mobility routine using a lacrosse ball. You can pick one up on Amazon for a few bucks.

Spend two to five minutes on each of these per side. It's OK for them to be uncomfortable, but they should not bring on your familiar back pain.

Plantar Fascia

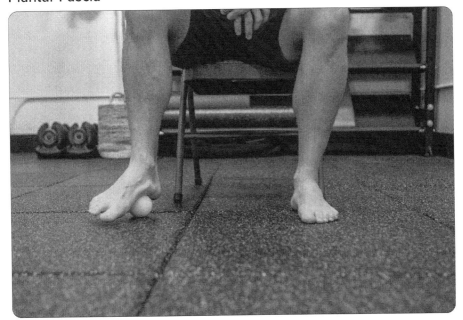

Calf

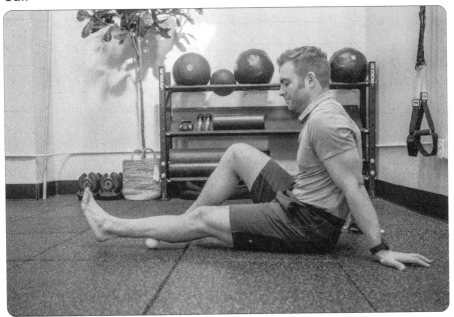

Shin

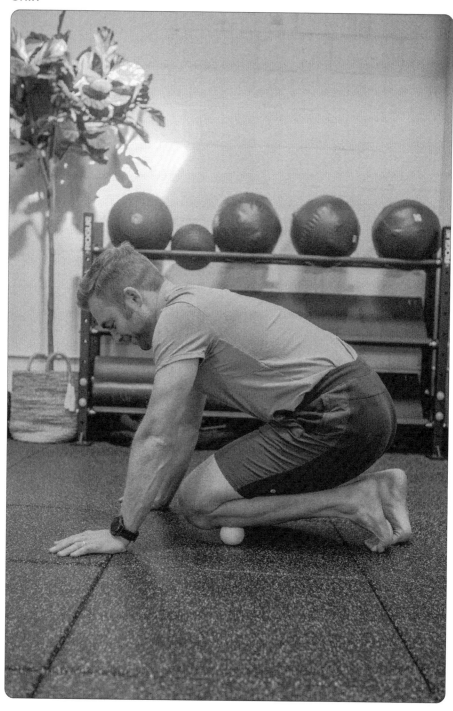

Outer Thigh

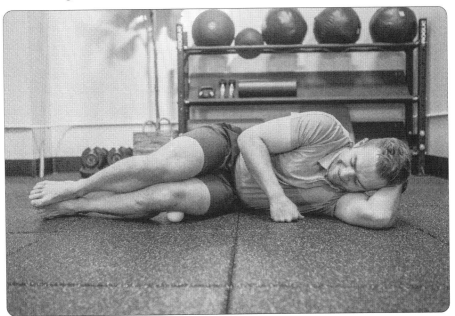

Tensor Fascia Lata

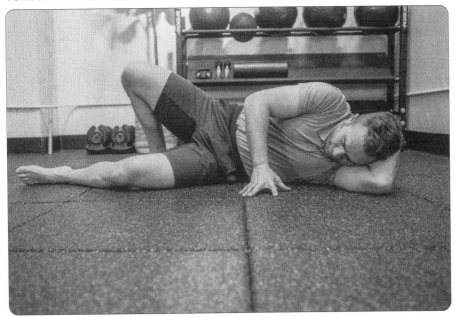

Hip Flexor

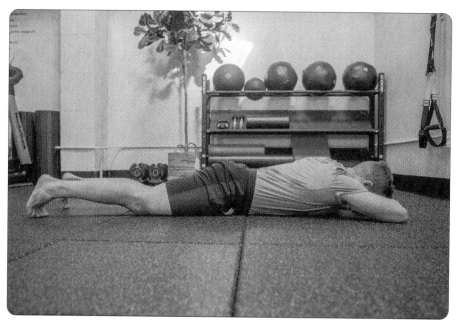

Glutes

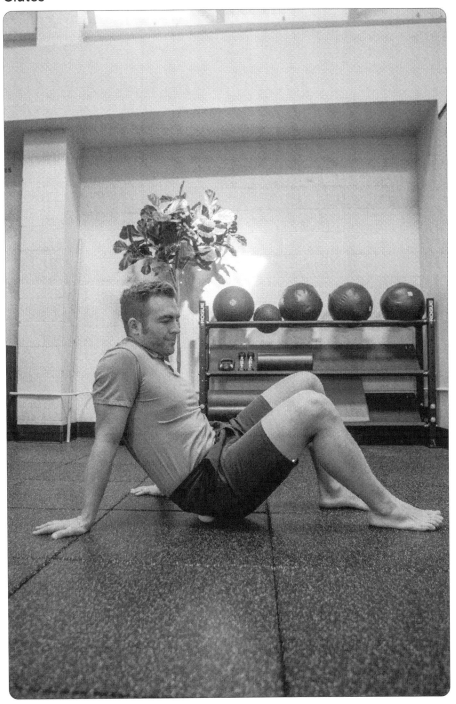

Low Back

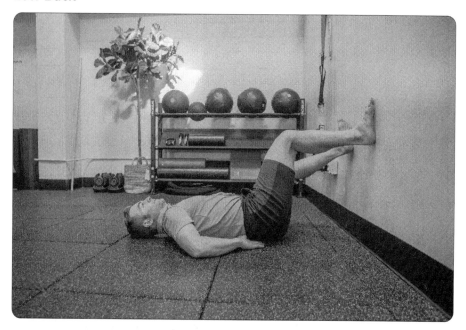

Upper Traps

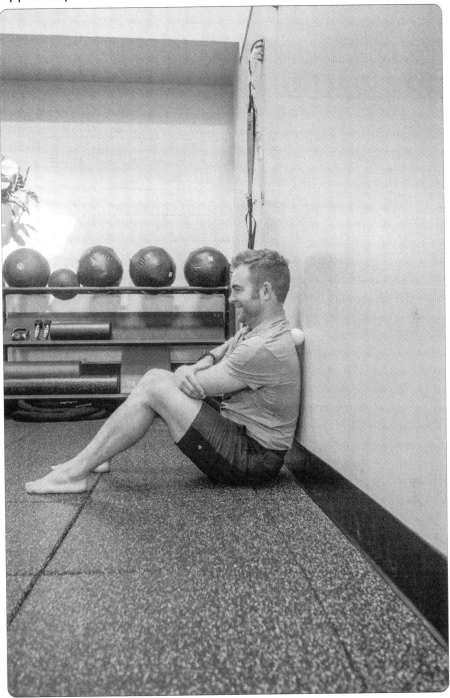

Chest

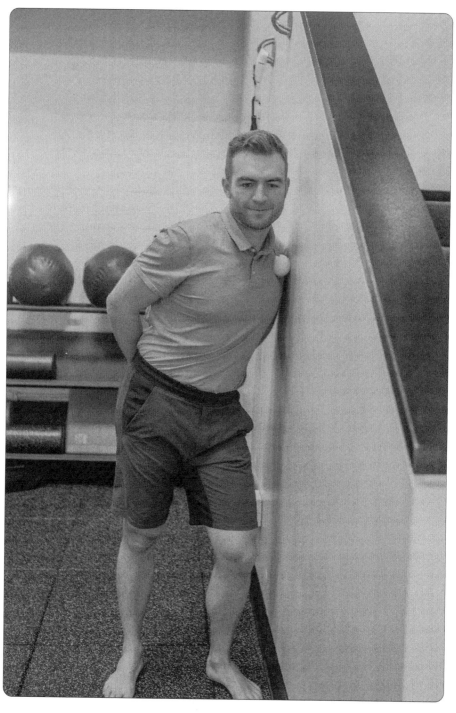

Neck

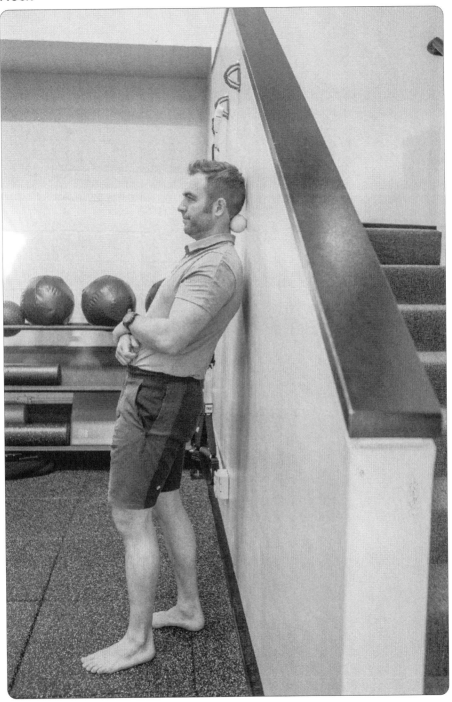

Hamstrings

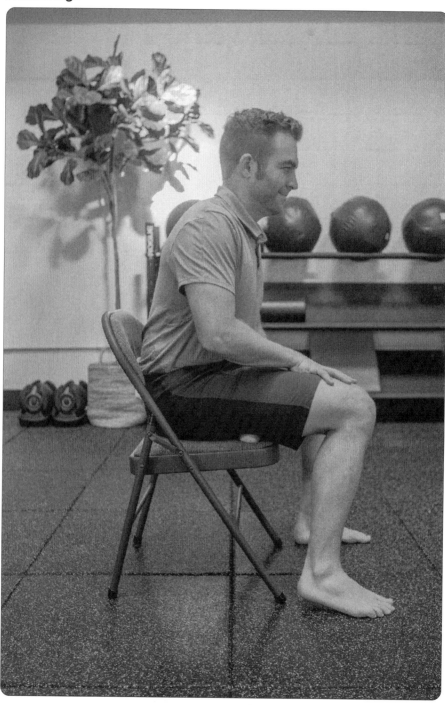

It Feels Pso-Rite

Some fitness implements are marketing gimmicks. Others, like the Pso-Rite, solve problems. 21st century humans sit way too much. Even if we exercise and balance out with a standing desk, our hip flexors are still likely to be tight. These muscles have attachments to our spine and can create compressive forces and make us more likely to have low back pain. Take 5 to 10 minutes a day to lay on the Pso-Rite and watch what it does for your back pain. Go gently at first, as this can be intense.

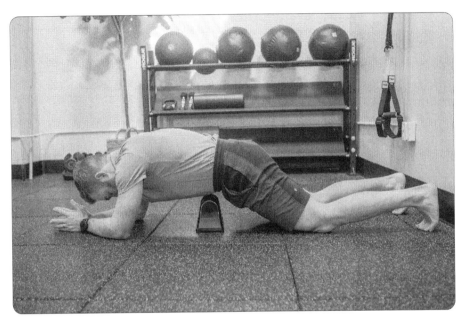

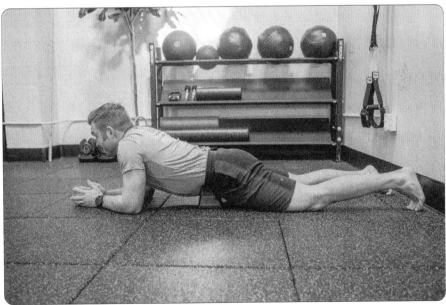

Foam Roller

You can use a foam roller for most of the mobilizations above with the lacrosse ball. However, a lacrosse can get deeper into tight muscles and is our recommendation.

But for an exercise like thoracic spine extension, you need something like a foam roller to get the leverage and height to extend your upper back.

Thoracic Spine Extension

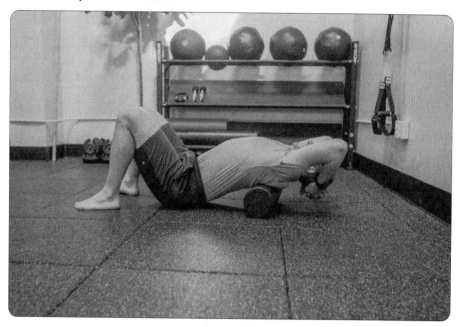

Stretches For Beating Back Pain

Extension

With all the sitting we do, most folks flex forward more than they extend backwards. But in order to walk and stand, we need extension. So give your back some extension love.

Start by simply laying on the ground for 5 to 10 minutes. You can even put a pillow under your belly if it's too painful. Then, slowly press yourself up higher and higher.

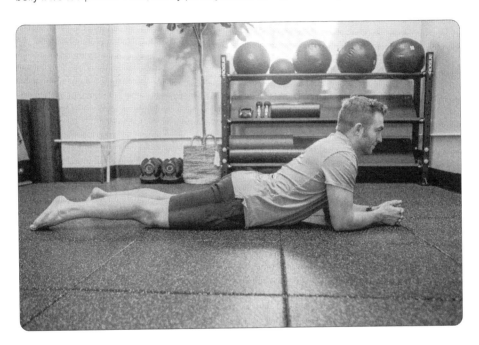

Eventually, you can push all the way up on your hands. Instead of holding this one for 5 to 10 minutes, perform 50 reps of chest all the way down and all the way up in 10 minutes.

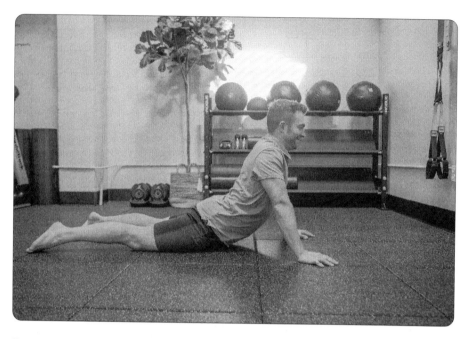

Then, take it up standing. Perform 50 in 10 minutes.

Chapter 8: Balls, Core, And Stretches Galore

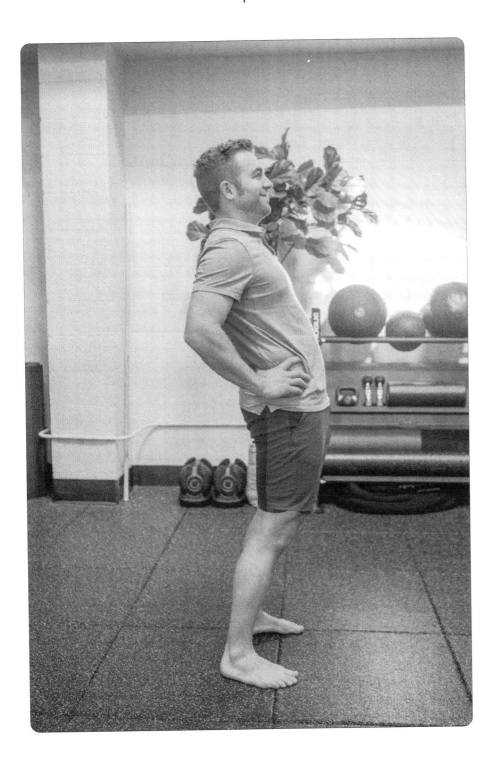

Last, for an advanced challenge, you can attempt a back bridge as pictured below. Shoot for 5 30-second holds in a span of 10 minutes.

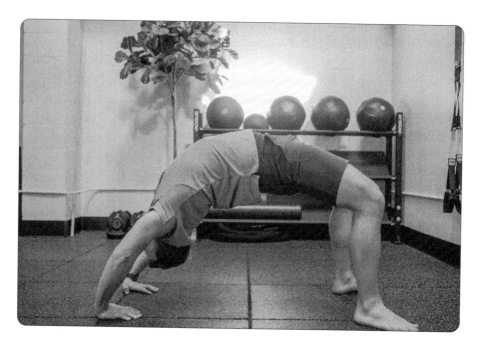

Calves and Ankles

Tightness in the calves and ankles can cause compensations all the way up to the lower back. So make sure you have good mobility. Try holding each of these stretches for 5 minutes per side.

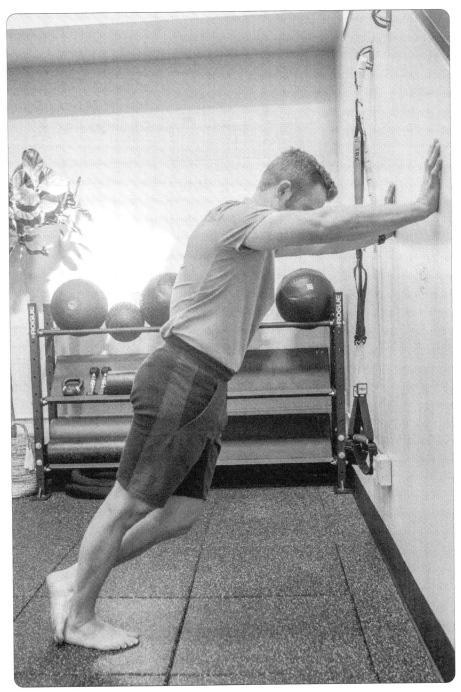

Bent Knee Ankle Stretch

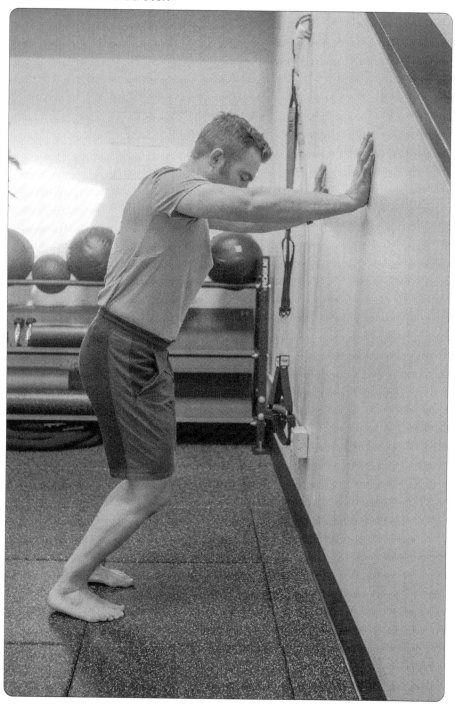

Pigeon

Give your piriformis and sciatica nerve some love with this stretch.

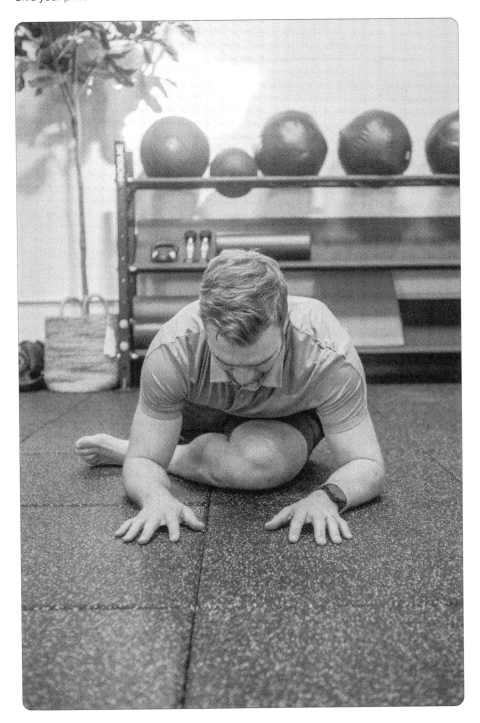

Hamstring Forward Bend

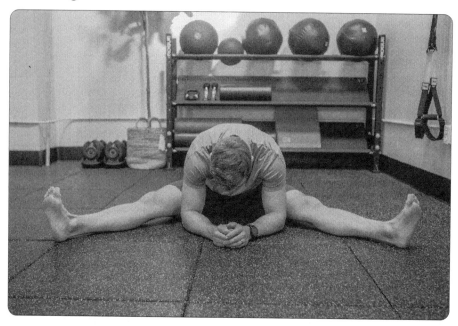

Down Dog Pedal

Gently pedal your feet up and down feeling a big stretch on the heel down leg side.

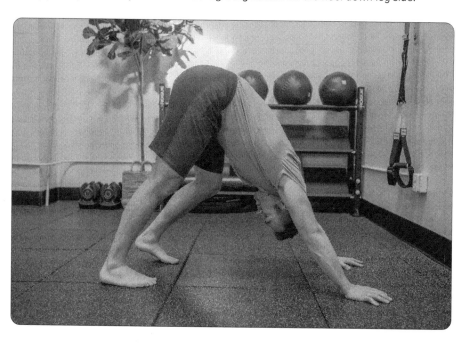

Hip Flexors Level 1

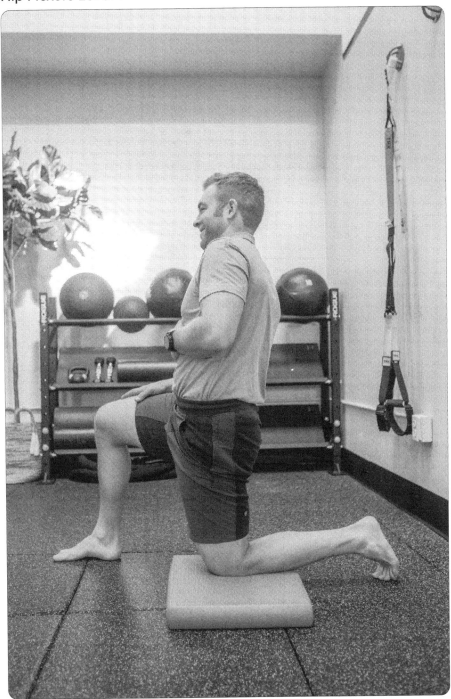

Hip Flexors Level 2

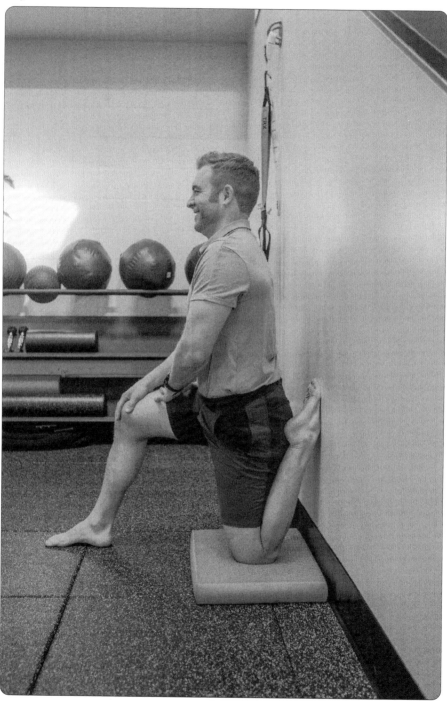

Butterfly

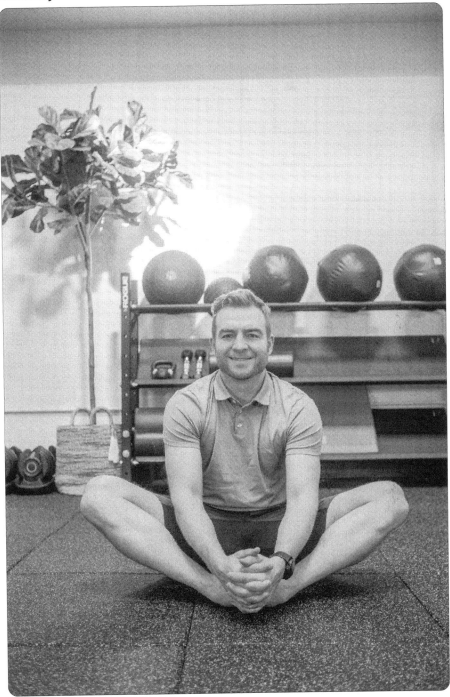

Band Stretches

You can snag a mobility band on Amazon.

Band-Assisted Squat

Wrap the band around your lower back. Slowly lower yourself down into a squat position. Hold for 2 to 5 minutes. You can shift your weight back and forth from foot to foot.

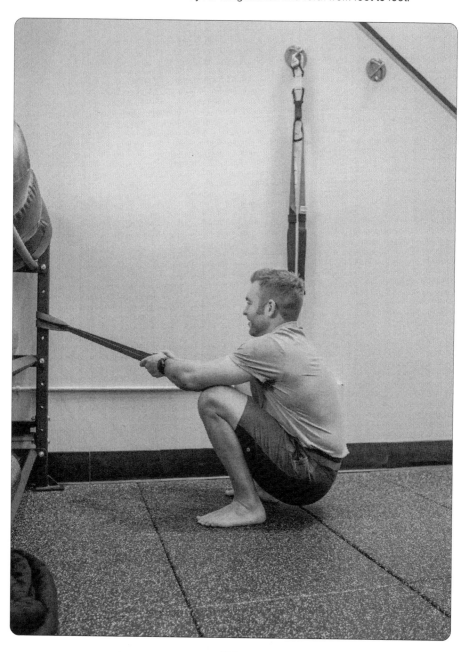

Band Down Dog Hip Stretch

With the band firmly secured to something immovable, wrap the other end around the front of one thigh. Reach your hands to the ground. You can alternate between bending and straightening out your knee of the leg that's on the ground.

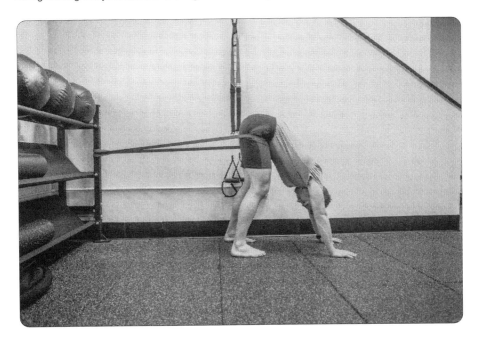

Half-Kneeling Band Stretch

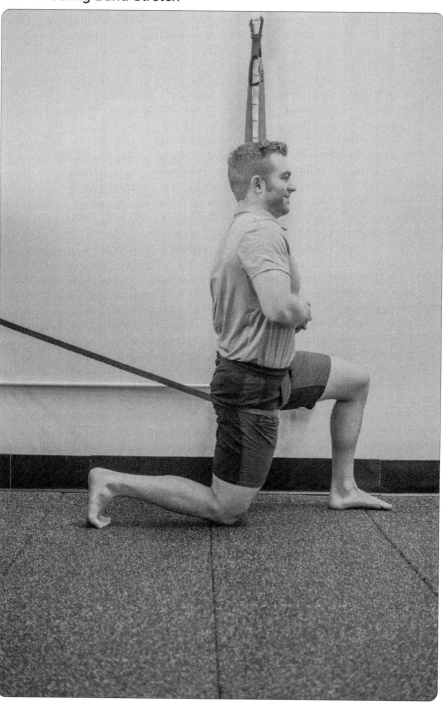

Band Shoulder Extension

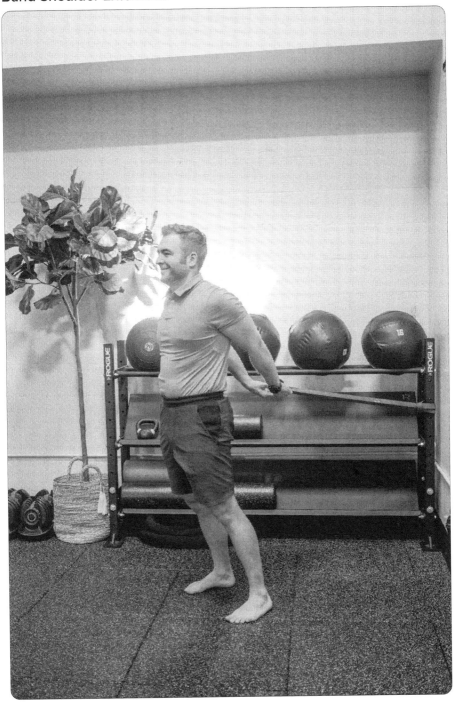

Band Overhead Shoulder Stretch

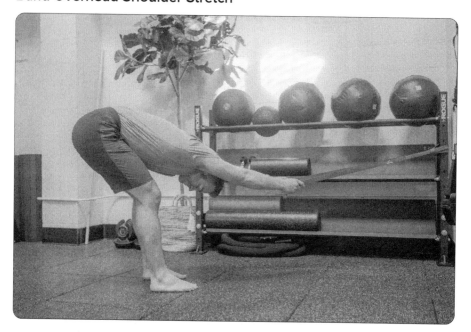

Back Pain Core Routine

How do you strengthen your core?

This is one of our most commonly asked questions. The truth about a really strong core is that the easiest way to get it is without doing any traditional "core exercises." No sit-ups. No crunches. No twists. In fact, many of these old-school core exercises actually damage discs. One of our patients had been doing 200 sit-ups a day for the last 30 years. We told him to stop, and by the next week, his back pain was already gone!

Instead of these types of exercises that focus on moving the trunk, a strong core is built by resisting movement at the trunk while generating movement at the limbs. To put that in context, during a deadlift, the hips move while the spine stays still. For another example, during a standing chest press, the arms move while the trunk remains still. In order for this to happen, the body needs to be free to support itself. Locking yourself into an exercise machine that stabilizes your whole body prevents you from actively resisting movement in your trunk because the machine does it for you. Think of it this way, if your trunk would move if not for your active, intentional resistance during an exercise, you're doing some killer core work.

Let's get to the core program!

Back Core Level 1

Before moving to Level 2, you should be able to hold each of these exercises for 60 seconds without back pain.

Side Plank With Bottom Knee Down

Lay on your side. Push through your bottom elbow and knee lifting your top hip towards the ceiling. Work up to holding this position for 60 seconds on each side without pain.

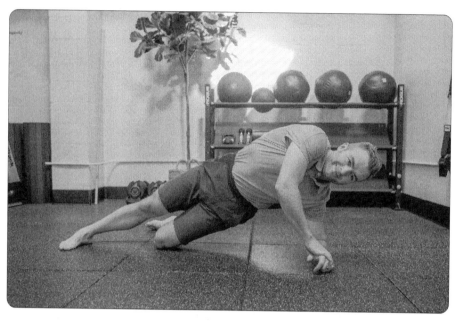

90-90 Hold

Lay on your back with your hips and knees bent at 90-degree angles. Keep your back firmly pressed into the ground. Breathe and hold.

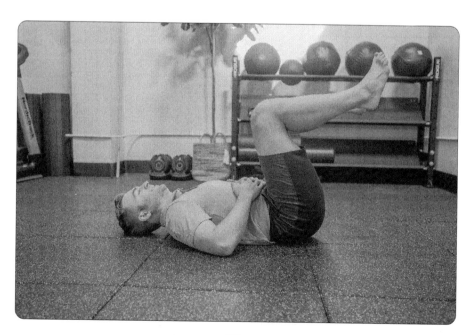

Modified Plank

With your knees on the ground, tuck your tail and lift your spine up towards the ceiling. Breathe and hold, working up to 60 seconds without back pain.

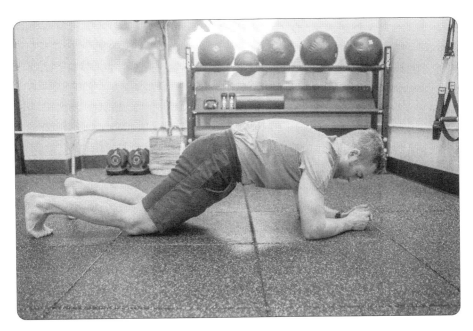

Back Core Level 2
Leg Lowers and Bicycles — Easy:

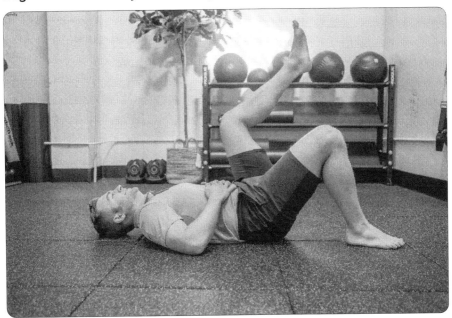

Leg Lowers and Bicycles — Medium:

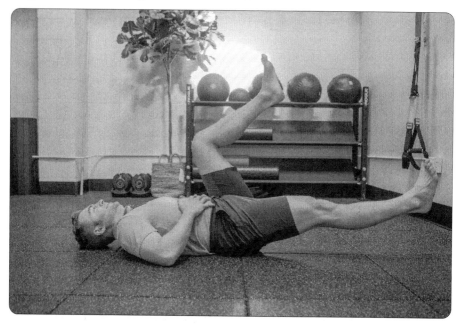

Leg Lowers and Bicycles — Hard:

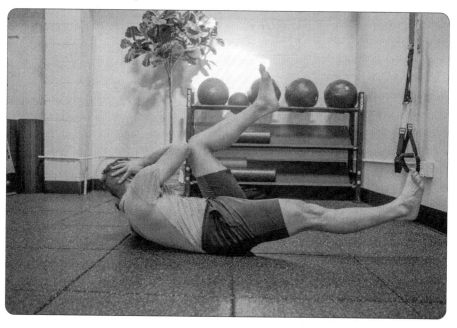

Side Plank

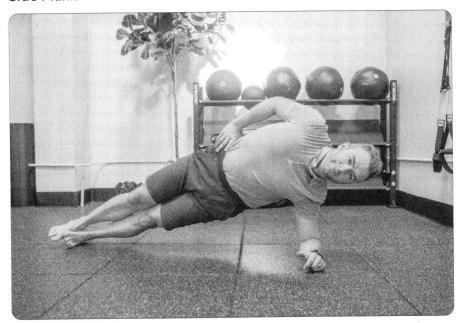

Plank

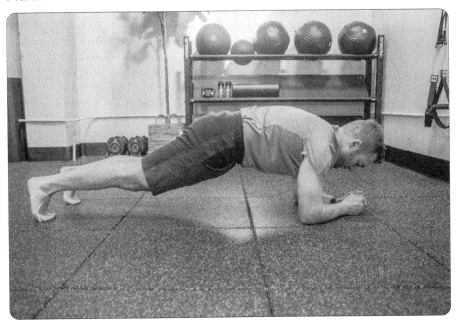

BONUS: Hollow Body Hold

Keeping your back firmly pressed into the ground, lower your hands and legs as close to the ground as possible. Once you can hold your legs and arms a few inches off the ground for a minute without back pain, you have achieved maximum bulletproofing of your core and spine.

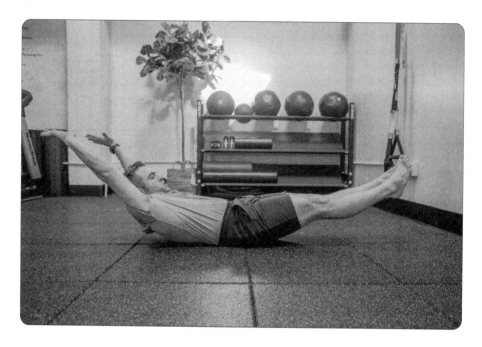

Part 3: The Principles

Chapter 9: The Village Principles

If you've been dealing with low back pain for months to years, chances are you've tried various treatments and didn't find permanent, lasting relief. That's why you're reading this book. Maybe you've tried taking pain pills, gotten injections, or even had a failed surgery. You're frustrated, worried about the future, but you haven't given up hope.

When you set out to solve a problem like easing back pain, you will inescapably reach a point where the only way forward is to do something different. After all, what you are really seeking is change, and how can things change if what you do is the same? But this point, this inevitable, pivotal point of choice always comes with a question. And that question is: "How do I know if this will work?"

This isn't just the big question our clients ask before they sign on the dotted line. It is the question we at Village pursue day after day after day. After all our years working with thousands of people just like you, we think we may have a start to the answer to that question. And the answer was right under our noses the whole time. It's you. You see, you came to us with problems, and we solved them together. You came to us with goals, and together we achieved them. Together we navigated the unknown, overcame setbacks, and ultimately felt the joy of a work accomplished. Through it all, we learned exactly which characteristics defined the most successful version of you.

These highly successful characteristics are named in the following 12 principles. They are full of old and new wisdom. Some are backed by irrefutable science. Others push boundaries. While it is always easier and safer to stay in the comfort zone of convention, it has become apparent that this comfort zone is a breeding ground for all sorts of modern illnesses. Low back pain, obesity, type 2 diabetes, dementia, arthritis, chronic pain, and the aftermath of pharmaceutical and surgical errors are choking our society of its life and liberty. We cannot stand by idly.

Note: We did not write these principles specifically for people with low back pain. Yet, implementing these 12 principles into your life will create an environment within your body where you are very unlikely to have low back pain. Furthermore, these principles extend beyond pain into other areas of health, like losing weight, managing inflammation, avoiding chronic diseases, and preserving your mental health.

Know this: Anyone can follow these principles, but following them will make you different. We live in a sick world — your vibrant health will stick out like a sore thumb. Sometimes people will praise you; sometimes they will mock you. If you are ready for this, you are ready for these principles. They are not so dogmatic as to micromanage your behavior, but they are specific enough to be understood and measured. These are the Village Principles.

Chapter 10: Control Carbs

Get ready for a fruit punch! You wouldn't start your day with a Pepsi and consider it healthy, yet breakfast plates filled with fruits are anything but nutritious. Like pugs, poodles, and the infamous labradoodle, healthy, genetically winning traits like strength and mental sanity were bred out of these dogs in favor of absolute cuteness. Similarly, everything that made fruits nutrient dense and immuno-protective has been lost in the quest for the sweetest, most eye-appealing specimens. Over the past several generations, food scientists have bred oranges, apples, bananas, and many other staples not for nutrient density but for sugar content and shelf life. Stack that with any of the other "heart-healthy, whole-grain" options as "part of a balanced breakfast" and you have a meal that is shockingly high in carbohydrates.

Wait, what? Heart-healthy grains aren't healthy?

Not really. Yes, you'll get a little fiber and a few vitamins, but the cumulative effect of a diet high in carbohydrates is the same as a diet high in sugar, because a diet high in carbohydrates IS a diet high in sugar. By the way, if you want to get that "heart-healthy" label slapped on your cereal box, all you need to do is send the American Heart Association a rather large check. It's branding. It's marketing. It's not nutrition.

This wasn't much of a problem a hundred years ago, because people's eating habits and active lifestyles were totally different from the modern American's. A hundred years ago, carbs were already under control. The modern American is under-rested, over-stressed, and inundated with advertising and food additives that drive excessive feeding. This type of excessive feeding leaves us particularly vulnerable to the effects of carbohydrates. While fats and proteins can be delicious, they don't have nearly the effect on our neurological reward system.

Why does this matter?

Even though we've been raised to believe that the sugars in fruits and the "complex carbohydrates" from grains are a healthy source of calories, the truth is that they are little better than that can of soda when it comes to their collective effect on our blood sugar, insulin response, waistline, and brain function.

Here's why:

Carbohydrates, regardless of their glycemic index, turn into sugar. That sugar goes to the bloodstream, upsets its delicate composition, and requires a rapid insulin response to literally prevent death by blood toxicity. To put it in perspective, at any given time we should only have a teaspoon of sugar in our entire six liters of blood. A single modern banana contains six teaspoons of sugar by the time it's digested. Insulin keeps us alive, but not without consequence. The problem with over demand of the insulin system is twofold. First, a system that is constantly flooded with insulin will eventually become insensitive, and this is what we call type 2 diabetes. Hopefully you don't need an explanation for why that is bad. Second, insulin can make us more susceptible to weight gain via its promotion of fat storage. This is because all the sugar removed from the bloodstream (to prevent us from dying) has to go somewhere. And you guessed it, it goes to storage as body fat.

Remember the balance of blood we were just talking about? In an environment inundated by carbohydrates, our blood vessels actually get sticky. That's right — the same way sugary foods make a toddler's hands a sticky mess, so it is with your arteries. This is a big issue because arteries need to be flexible and adaptable. They are covered in a layer of smooth muscle that helps them regulate blood pressure and blood flow so that your body can perform optimally in all types of situations, whether lying down for a nap or "laying up" for two points in a pickup basketball game. Over time, carbohydrate molecules bind with proteins on the surface of your arteries, causing them to be rigid and sticky. Believe it or not, the scientific term for these bonds is "advanced glycation end products," or AGEs. Carbs literally AGE your blood vessels!

While most folks are afraid of cholesterol-causing arterial plaques, it is really the assaults against the integrity of the arterial wall such as AGEs that set us up for vascular failure.

Chronic high-carb consumption also contributes to high levels of systemic inflammation. Every chronic disease known to man has been linked to inflammation. Alzheimer's, heart disease, cancer, and even Parkinson's all have a bevy of research linking them to inflammation.

Alright, so we've got your attention and you want to get control of your carbs. But what do you eat? Many clients we work with begin to go through their day and wonder how they will get enough calories from the food they are eating. Ubiquitous staples like oatmeal for breakfast, turkey on wheat for lunch, and spaghetti for dinner all contribute to overconsumption of carbs. Instead, imagine a delicious egg and vegetable scramble for breakfast, a beautiful fresh salad for lunch with avocados and lemon vinaigrette, and a petite ribeye with herbs and asparagus for dinner. Throw in a few nuts, seeds, berries, and a probiotic-rich yogurt or pickle here and there and you've got everything your body needs. Just to be clear, this is not a "Keto" diet because the body is not going into ketosis. Neither is it Atkins. We wouldn't even call this a low-carb, high-fat (LCHF) diet. We would consider it a historically accurate average carb diet. However, that does not have a ring to it, so for now, it will be unnamed!

Chapter 11: Eat Healthy Fats

Let's talk about healthy fats... "Wait, WHAT? Healthy and fat can't go together, right?"

They can!

Despite decades of misinformation about fat, the truth is finally coming out. Even the CDC has finally started talking about healthy fats.[16]

To understand why natural fats can be so healthy, let's first talk about what they do in the body. Second, let's address a few common myths. Last, let's talk about how to integrate healthy fats into your diet.

Fats play key roles in multiple body systems. They provide clean, sustainable energy that doesn't peak and crash like a carb-based diet. They provide the primary matter for brain tissue, composing about 60% of its total mass. They are the lipids of the remarkable phospholipid-bilayer that allows every single one of our trillions of cells to have a functioning boundary between itself and its neighbors. They provide the critical insulation to our electric-wire-like nerves known as myelin. They allow the storage of vitamins A, D, E, and K. They provide substance for cholesterol, which is critical in hormonal regulation. Omega-3 fatty acids are one of the most powerful anti-inflammatories around, curbing pain and boosting immunity. And so much more!

An exhaustive list of everything that fat does in the body would be quite long because fats are necessary in virtually all physiological processes. But if fat is so essential to life, why is it vilified?

In fact, the attack on fat is only a recent cultural phenomenon. Throughout human history, fat has been a sought-after commodity. The change occurred after Ancel Keys' famous Seven Countries Study conducted from 1958 to 1978. What followed was an unprecedented shift in public policy and medical perspective that led to an even more unprecedented shift in human behavior.

To give context, you have to understand that food is one of the primary elements of

---

16 "Healthy Eating Tips | DNPAO | CDC." https://www.cdc.gov/nccdphp/dnpao/features/national-nutrition-month/index.html. Accessed 30 Apr. 2020.

human culture. What we eat and how we eat it is a profound representation of our natural resources, social habits, and even religious values. Today, the research of Ancel Keys and his contemporaries is hotly debated. We won't delve into that debate here, only suggest that a rapid departure from traditional food should merit extraordinary, irrefutable evidence. The only fat with this type of damning evidence is trans fat, which, ironically, is still being snuck into tons of "diet" and "healthy" foods as mono- and diglycerides. You can't make this stuff up.

It gets worse. Once touted as healthy alternatives to traditional fats, the industrial seed oils like canola, corn, cottonseed, soy, safflower, sunflower, and their kin have demonstrably inflammatory effects in the body. So, what to do?

Eat real, healthy fats. The kinds of fats that humans have always eaten — not the processed stuff in boxed foods, nor the designer, "heart-healthy" margarine tubs, nor the chemically altered versions of various cash crops. Avoid the stuff from maltreated feedlot animals. Choose fresh, unrefined oils of organic plants and seeds that are actually oily (think avocados, almonds, olives, and similar). Choose fresh, pasture-raised, 100% grass-fed, wild-caught, organic animals and dairy products.

Healthy fats aren't just a cleaner, more evenly burning fuel source for your body. They provide critical roles in virtually every physiological system. More relevant than ever are their essential roles in immune function. They help us heal from a myriad of internal and external injuries while simultaneously preventing future sickness, chronic pain, and degeneration of our joints, arteries, and brain tissue.

Now put down your 0% Greek yogurt and your fat-free, high-sugar salad dressing and eat some delicious, pan-seared salmon!

Chapter 12: Prioritize Veggies

Since the dawn of the human race, vegetation has been the foundation of the food chain. We foraged for vegetables and hunted animals that grazed on vegetables. Abruptly, around the time of the agricultural revolution, our eating patterns changed for the worse. Fast forward to present day, and nearly 70% of the caloric intake worldwide comes from grains, sugars, and toxic fats.[17] This shift in nutrients and calories has not been without consequence. Even with advances in modern medicine, it's projected that by the year 2031, HALF of the U.S. population will be classified as chronically ill.[18]

Consuming five or more servings of vegetables per day drastically reduces our risk of chronic inflammatory diseases.[19] Intuitively, we know vegetable consumption is vital. Yet less than 10% of Americans consume the recommended five-plus servings of vegetables per day.[20] Why is it so difficult?

The answer is inside each of us. In our head, to be exact. We have a brain that is inclined towards the instantly gratifying instead of what's best long term. Society today is happy to quench our thirst for a quick hit of dopamine (the feel-good hormone) with sugar, cheap grains, toxic oils, Netflix, and Facebook. Vegetables, like most good things in life, take time, effort, and don't instantly appease the reward centers in our noggins. Furthermore, people today are over-busy, stressed, and leave little time to prepare vegetables. And when we do make veggies, they are usually tasteless, out of season, over-cooked mush. It's no wonder it's so difficult to abide by mom's advice to "eat your vegetables." So, how do we prioritize veggies and make them more frequent fare on our dinner plates?

A paradigm shift is in order. Instead of thinking of vegetables as a small side to our main course of grains and meat, they need to become the centerpiece. Let's take a staple on most Americans' weekly dinner menu: Pasta with red sauce. For many, that is already the whole dish. A step in the right direction adds a high-quality meat or protein. Even fewer will bother with a vegetable. If they do, it's probably an afterthought, often as inconsequential as

---

17 "What the World Eats | National Geographic." https://www.nationalgeographic.com/what-the-world-eats/. Accessed 27 Apr. 2020.
18 "Percentage of the Population With Chronic Diseases, 1995 ...." https://www.silverbook.org/fact/percentage-of-the-population-with-chronic-diseases-1995-2030/. Accessed 27 Apr. 2020.
19 "Disparities in State-Specific Adult Fruit and Vegetable ... - CDC." https://www.cdc.gov/mmwr/volumes/66/wr/mm6645a1.htm. Accessed 27 Apr. 2020.
20 "Disparities in State-Specific Adult Fruit and Vegetable ... - CDC." https://www.cdc.gov/mmwr/volumes/66/wr/mm6645a1.htm. Accessed 27 Apr. 2020.

a little frozen spinach thrown into the sauce. But what if that spinach was the backbone of the dish? Imagine a plate full of spinach sauteed in herbed butter. In the center of the plate, a small clearing where a delicate nest of noodles and red sauce cradles a trio of homestyle meatballs. Nutrient-dense. Satisfying. And most importantly, allows you to enjoy a few extra special bites of pasta rather than gorging yourself into a bottomless pasta pit.

Now that your mouth is watering, let's break down this fantasy dish a little. The most important part is rethinking proportions so that vegetables are featured while the other elements are highlighted. Highlighting every line in a book would be pointless, and so is covering your entire plate in carbs. Second, the spinach in our fantasy dish was cooked in... butter! Yum!

Like a friend who tells us the truth even when it hurts, veggies need a little help to bring out their best. Instead of the truth when we need to hear it, veggies need fat, heat, and salt to achieve their full potential. Not only do veggies taste bland when cooked without salt and fat, but they are also less nutritious. Cooking vegetables breaks down the plants' cell walls, releasing otherwise locked-up nutrients. Using a healthy fat and good sea salt coaxes flavor ligands and phytonutrients in contact with our taste buds AND makes nutrients available to us in our bloodstream.

This is wonderful news! It means that you can light up the reward centers in your brain when you eat vegetables rather than choke them down out of sheer will power. Psychologically, eating veggies becomes an effortless habit rather than a major chore. Sharpen up your knife skills a little and it won't be long before you are throwing all kinds of veggies into breakfast, lunch, and dinner. It's a brave new world, and veggies are back on the menu!

You can do better than the side salad. Iceberg lettuce (and most other tasteless lettuces) have very little nutritional value. Most pre-packaged salad dressings contain toxic fats, food additives, and high levels or sugar (or fake sugar). Your best bet is to make your own salad at home with dark, leafy greens, a plethora of other veggies, a liberal pour of olive oil, and a splash of balsamic vinegar.

Believe it or not, there are real humans who are mind-blowingly passionate about things like soil, ecosystems, and vegetables. And they live in little tarp-covered booths in farmers markets around the country for a few hours each week. OK, OK, they live in regular houses (sometimes farm houses). Go talk to them. Ask them what you should buy and what you should cook. Ask them how you can make better decisions about produce. These agricultural heroes are treasure troves of knowledge, and if we don't get to know them and buy their stuff, they will go away and we will be left with endless fields of genetically modified cash crops.

Most people never consider that quality produce benefits them without ever being on their plate. Why? Fruits and vegetables are symbols of our land, and our land is our livelihood. When you allocate your resources towards quality produce, you create economic demand for healthy soil and balanced ecosystems. When our land is well cared for, everything (including

Chapter 12: Prioritize Veggies

people you've never met) are better off. Don't be fooled by false frugality! Investing in healthy environments across the board pays dividends for generations to come. In the process, you'll create an environment of health for yourself and your family.

Chapter 13: Source Responsibly

Does the sourcing of our animal products matter? It's time to put a "steak" in the ground with an emphatic "yes!"

Your body is like an eager student at a fascinating TED Talk sitting on the edge of his seat, furiously taking notes. The "information" in this TED Talk comes in the form of the environment we live in — information like vitamin D from sun exposure, hormonal balance from deep rest, spikes of cortisol from a stressful conflict left unresolved, a boost in immunity from an appropriate workout, or nutritional communication from our food. The notes that the body writes are the expression of our genetic code. Will we be healthy or progress towards disease? The answer is determined in large part by our environment.[21]

To have a healthy body, you can't communicate with it using chemical-ladden, factory-produced, and feedlot foods. You want blue skies, green pastures, and happy, healthy animals behaving according to their genetic code. After all, eating is taking something from the outside world, putting it inside your body, and letting your body make it part of who you are. That's right — you are what you eat!

A very tangible way the environment of our food impacts us is the omega-3 to omega-6 ratio. The balance of omega-3:6 fatty acids in our diet may be the most important ratio to manage for avoiding diseases linked to chronic inflammation like heart disease, cancer, and alzheimers.[22] The ideal is a ratio of 1:1 to 1:4. The average american today trends towards 1:20.[23] Omega-6s are like the gas pedal for the immune and inflammatory process. Omega-3s are like the brakes. Imagine trying to drive to work in a Corvette with no brakes. It's a recipe for disaster and disease.[24] 100% grass-fed meat has close to a 1:1 ratio of omega-3:6, whereas grain-fed meat is closer to 1:15. This is due to grains being high in omega-6 fatty acids and greens being balanced.

But isn't meat bad for us? The "scientific" research cited by shockingly titled articles like

---

[21] "Defining the Environment in Gene–Environment ... - NCBI - NIH." https://www.ncbi.nlm.nih.gov/pmc/articles/PMC3786759/. Accessed 30 Apr. 2020.
[22] "Omega-3 fatty acids in health and disease and in growth and ...." https://www.ncbi.nlm.nih.gov/pubmed/1908631. Accessed 30 Apr. 2020.
[23] "An Increase in the Omega-6/Omega-3 Fatty ...." 2 Mar. 2016, https://www.ncbi.nlm.nih.gov/pmc/articles/PMC4808858/. Accessed 30 Apr. 2020.
[24] "Health Implications of High Dietary Omega-6 ... - NCBI." 5 Apr. 2012, https://www.ncbi.nlm.nih.gov/pmc/articles/PMC3335257/. Accessed 30 Apr. 2020.

"meat causes cancer"[25] tends to come from studies[26] that use feedlot meats cooked in toxic oils and make universal claims about all animal products. The truth is most red meat is poorly sourced and is paired with toxins. The burger from In-N-Out cooked in vegetable oil and placed in between a bun made from cheap grains is a far cry from the 100% grass-fed steak cooked in a stable cooking oil like avocado oil that we encourage our clients to consume.

Choosing well sourced animal products is also better for the environment, the economy, and the animal.

Nobody looks at an idyllic, green pastureland with scattered animals grazing and thinks, "Yeah, that's disgusting. That definitely needs to be converted into a dusty, industrial ranch complex." People drive out of their way to take the "scenic route" through pasturelands! There's something about it that is good for the soul, and we recognize it even if we can't explain why. When we buy and consume animal products from animals in their natural environment, we promote the preservation and stewardship of these wide-open spaces. But it's not just us and the animals that it benefits. These environments are mini-ecosystems that play host to hundreds of other creatures. The alternative industrial ranch complex? Not so much.

The meat and dairy industries are big business with big government lobbyists ensuring the people at the top are making big salaries. However, the average farmer is working in less than ideal conditions, has little control over his own farm, and is grossly underpaid. This pushes away talented and passionate farmers and leaves most of the work to less skilled hands. Instead of an artisanal craft, meat and dairy production become one more cog in the economic wheel that steamrolls over the livelihood of farmers and well-being of consumers.

If you are used to paying $3 for a pound of ground beef, you may need to rethink the true cost. While 100% grass-fed meat from a good source is significantly more expensive, it is not an apples-to-apples comparison. Currently, a pound of 100% grass-fed beef can be as much as $10 to $13 per pound. That's a tough deal to swallow for folks used to buying ground beef for $3 per pound. Similarly, pasture-raised eggs and wild-caught fish command a premium price. But besides paying for actual nutrients, enzymes, and probiotic content (not to mention better flavor), you are also paying towards fair wages for skilled farmers and the maintenance of our nation's most precious natural resource: land. That is a seriously worthy investment. The alternative is paying for the bonuses of agribusiness CEOs who care more about their bottom lines than their farmers, animals, or fields. As the old adage goes, "You get what you pay for." Additionally, when you have precious perishable food, you are much more likely to plan your days around eating it. It builds in motivation to resist drive-thru temptation. Dead food might last forever, but living beings need living foods.

---

25 "Even moderate red and processed meat eaters …." https://www.cancerresearchuk.org/about-us/cancer-news/press-release/2019-04-17-even-moderate-red-and-processed-meat-eaters-at-risk-of-bowel-cancer/. Accessed 23 Sept. 2020.
26 "Diet and colorectal cancer in UK Biobank: a prospective study." https://academic.oup.com/ije/article/49/1/246/5470096/. Accessed 23 Sept. 2020.

Chapter 13: Source Responsibly

Animals not given antibiotics and toxic chemicals have to be extremely well taken care of. They cannot be sick. They cannot be dirty. They cannot be crowded. This is in stark contrast to the average feedlot animal, which is guaranteed to be sick, dirty, and crowded. Their mistreatment is blanketed over by antibiotics and pasteurization. Antibiotics prevent dirty, crowded animals from dropping dead before they lose their economic value. Pasteurization prevents any pathogens present in milk due to suboptimal conditions from making it to consumers and extends its shelf life. But wouldn't it be better to just have healthy animals and healthy milk?

Creating cultural change is not easy. It feels "normal" to shop and eat the way we do when everyone around us is doing the same thing. It can feel extravagant or excessive to pay more for food, especially if you were raised to believe that frugality is a moral virtue. But if we want to be healthy and vote for change with our dollars, we must choose well sourced animal products.

Chapter 14: Rest Deeply

How is a successful human like a slingshot? It's simple: If we want to shoot far in life, we need to put ourselves under tension, then let go. For most of you reading this, putting yourself under tension is not a problem. You've worked hard, taken on lots of responsibilities, and generally said yes to whatever life asks of you. Between your career, family, and that random volunteering gig you agreed to again, your schedule is full. The tension is there!

But what happens when a slingshot gets pulled farther and farther back without ever being released? Well, it snaps! As paradoxical as it seems, the real key to getting ahead is allowing yourself to let go, to rest deeply.

Today, we feel an overwhelming pressure to do everything. To be everything to everyone. In order to be "successful," we need to wake up before dawn to exercise, work a full-time job all day, and be a full-time parent at night. We need to take our kids to every single activity (will they still get into a good college if they don't play all the sports and do all the activities?).

When we do "rest," we're bad at it. Instead of disconnecting from technology and engaging with nature, sleeping deeply, or conversing with loved ones, we sit in front of screens to numb our minds or compare ourselves to others on social media.

First, let's talk about sleep. In a typical 24-hour period, the human body goes through a complex sequence of hormone cascades also known as a circadian rhythm. Our energy level, sleepiness, hunger, bathroom habits, metabolism, immune system, and mental clarity are all the product of delicately metered hormone releases. Whether we submit or rebel against this rhythm will determine much of our potential for health or for disease. We are meant to sleep when it's dark, wake naturally with the light of dawn, and spend time outside each day. If we stay up late watching Netflix or scrolling Facebook, wake up hours before first light to an alarm and spend all day inside, we create a confusing slew of unnatural hormonal changes inside our body.

But rest isn't just about sleep. We tell our bodies to enter an environment of rest or stress with food, movement, conversations, and how we breathe.

When we eat sugar, grains, vegetable oil, alcohol, and a depressingly long list of common food additives, we thrust our bodies into fight-or-flight mode as they quarrel with the onslaught of incoming toxins. Conversely, when we eat foods that communicate well with our bodies like nutrient-dense veggies, healthy fats, and well sourced animal products, we give our bodies the building blocks to repair and regenerate.

When we engage in chronic cardio activities at moderate to high intensities like jogging, cycling classes, or intense boot camps, we create a taxing stress that can throw us out of rest mode for days. Yet, the right exercise in the right amounts can help make us more restful. Strength training, short but intense intervals, and tons of low-level movement like walking and hiking create an environment of health within our bodies.

Modern communication technology has the two-edged effect of allowing us connection to people all around the world while also tempting us to never unplug our delicate attention and decision capacities. Over consumption of technology has been linked with depression, anxiety, expectations of instant gratification, trouble focusing, a sense of isolation, obesity, neck pain, and even vision loss.[27] The average American takes one week or less of vacation per year. Yet even on vacation, we still check emails and work.

So, you're ready to rest deeply and let the slingshot go?

The first step towards creating a life of rest is to take control of what you can. You can't control your toddler waking up in the middle of the night, but you can create boundaries between work and home. You can't control the increasing pervasiveness of technology, but you can turn off your phone at 8 p.m. each night to converse with your spouse and read a book. Many of the constraints that we foist on ourselves as things we "have to do" are self-imposed. So take a vacation without checking your work email, feel free to say "no thanks" to the obligatory volunteering gig, and don't feel pressure to commit to the third simultaneous activity for your kid.

When you prioritize rest, you'll allow yourself to be the best version of you in every area of life that's important. If we want to maximize our potential to love well, to be healthy and fit, to raise kids well, to create meaningful work, and to leave a legacy, we have to let go of the slingshot from time to time. So pull back. Work hard. Exercise. Be intentional. And then let go. Rest deeply. You'll be amazed at how far you'll fly forward from this seemingly paradoxical action.

---

27   "Health and Technology - Digital ...." http://www.digitalresponsibility.org/health-and-technology. Accessed 12 May. 2020.

Chapter 15: Get Outside

Your idea of roughing it may be staying at a hotel with no room service. Your idea of unplugging may be visiting a coffee shop with no Wi-Fi. Not everyone needs to boat down the Amazon river or climb Mount Everest. But if you want to lead a healthy, productive life, you can't do it all in the great indoors. You've got to get outside! A little sun on the skin, a little fresh air in the lungs, a little sand between the toes can do a lot more good than most modern folks realize. Science backs this up.[28] Conversely, a little too much screen time, a little too much indoor pollution, a little too much comfort can silently sap your health.

Getting outside benefits virtually every system in your body. Here's just a brief snapshot of what happens:

First of all, it gets us looking at things that are far away. This changes how the muscles in our eyes behave. Looking at something far away after spending hours and hours up close with walls and screens is like your eyeballs stretching their legs after a long car ride. The longer you stay in the car, the more likely your legs and low back will cramp up. Tension headaches are often caused by similar mechanisms in the muscles that support eye movement and focus, including muscles in the upper neck and skull.

Second, real light from the sky helps us regulate our circadian rhythms. Sunny blue skies and peaceful glowing sunsets communicate profoundly with our hormones and neurotransmitters to promote deep sleep and energetic wakefulness. Replace it with an endless barrage of LEDs and our bodies get confused.

Third, modest amounts of sunlight interact with our skin to help our bodies produce vitamin D. Vitamin D is notoriously hard to regulate with nutrition and/or supplements, but get out in the sun and the body knows what to do.

Fourth, good bacteria in healthy ecosystems help communicate with good bacteria in our bodies. We are not made to live in sterile environments. At some point, modern humans became convinced that every surface we touch should be bleached and sterilized. The absence of bacteria can actually be just as harmful as an environment full of bad bacteria. The real trick is to expose your body to the bacteria in healthy ecosystems. Don't go drinking

---

[28] "Vitamin D and Depression: Where is all the ... - NCBI - NIH." https://www.ncbi.nlm.nih.gov/pmc/articles/PMC2908269/. Accessed 27 May. 2020.

the water from an LA aqueduct. Do go out to a national park or similar protected area and be an advocate for these places before they're all gone. Additionally, an organic home garden is a great place to create your own healthy ecosystem, complete with healthy bacteria. Get your hands dirty!

Fifth, when it comes to indoor air quality, it's hard to beat the power of an open window and a breeze. You might think that your carpets, walls, and furniture don't matter. The dust they shed is certainly not as bad as asbestos, but that doesn't mean it's completely inert. Of course, most of us intuitively know we feel better after something as simple as "getting some fresh air." So, why do we spend so much time inside and immersed in technology?

It's simple. We prefer a sense of control and consistency to a sense of wonder and trust. We feel safe around doors that we can lock. We feel comfortable in air that is climate and humidity controlled. We feel powerful in man-made environments because, well, we made them.

There's nothing wrong with spending our time in places we've made more hospitable, but we must not lose what the world beyond our buildings offers us. There is a reason we have phrases like "the sky's the limit" and "professional ceiling." If we want to be interesting, innovative people, we must take breaks from our ceilings and spend time under the infinite sky.

We are losing our connection with the natural world. Kids chop down trees in Minecraft instead of climbing them. In Yosemite, you'll behold teenagers with their heads buried in their cell phones instead of looking up at the mountains. Adults live, work, and even exercise indoors. As technology has advanced and beckoned us to stay glued to screens, our well-being has deteriorated.[29] Yet, when we get outside and connect with nature, we see an immediate positive impact on our mood and health.[30]

There is a growing misconception that it's cleaner and safer to stay inside, that the sun instantly causes skin cancer, and that all bacteria cause disease. The truth is quite the contrary. We often pollute our indoor environments without realizing it. Just think about asbestos. It's not hard to imagine that in 20 years we'll be ripping something else out of half our buildings that was discovered to be toxic. Our bodies receive vital communication from the rays of the sun, the air across our face from a steady breeze, and dirt directly on our feet. Connection with nature can help alleviate depression and anxiety. So, do yourself a favor: Get outside!

---

29 "More Time on Technology, Less Happiness? Associations ...." 22 May. 2019, https://journals.sagepub.com/doi/abs/10.1177/0963721419838244. Accessed 6 May. 2020.
30 "Spending at least 120 minutes a week in ...." 13 Jun. 2019, https://www.nature.com/articles/s41598-019-44097-3. Accessed 6 May. 2020.

Chapter 16: Solve Pain

Before we delve into the intricacies of pain, please note that we covered this Village Principle in depth in previous chapters.

Since infancy we learn that our world can hurt us. We learn that we can skin knees, bump heads, and even feel painful tears when we are left out or angry. We learn that some of our hurts heal while others linger. Sometimes we even experience pain so profoundly that it alters the course of our lives. Chances are you know someone whose pain led them to drastic choices, like leaving a job, a marriage, or even their religion. You probably know even more people who have pursued risky surgeries or developed dependencies to medications aimed at reducing pain. Yet, despite its ubiquity, few understand what pain actually is.

Take a moment and try to define it. Is it a feeling? Is it a signal? Is it physical? Emotional? Is it good? Bad? Helpful or harmful?

It is remarkably hard to put in a box. It's complex. It's often many things at once. While understanding WHAT pain is can be elusive, understanding HOW pain works is tremendously helpful. In fact, it can decrease the level of pain you feel.[31]

First and most importantly, you need to understand that pain is about danger and not damage.

You see, our bodies are hard-wired to protect themselves from damage BEFORE it happens. Imagine a car alarm that only went off after the car was stolen and long gone. That would be useless! To be effective, a good alarm must go off at the first hint of danger.

Think of security at LAX. If somebody sees a cloud of smoke, security is not going to wait to uncover the source of it before they take measures to ensure travelers' safety. Whether the smoke is coming from an actual fire or from a toaster in the employee lounge, all or part of the airport is going to get shut down. Our body's alarm system is no different. Sometimes the alarm system can be a little too... alarming!

You might be thinking, "OK, but what about when I know there is actual damage — when I can see that I've broken a bone or cut my skin?" Great question!

---

[31] "Pain is Weird: A Volatile, Misleading Sensation - Pain Science." 26 Aug. 2018, https://www.painscience.com/articles/pain-is-weird.php. Accessed 27 Sep. 2018.

Nobody likes to go to the doctor and get a needle stick. However, for some people, that little pin is a minor nuisance. For others, it is absolutely excruciating. It's not because people have different nerves. It's because people have different minds.

If the pain we feel when we get a needle stick was a communication of damage, it would be pretty mild for everyone. However, because it is a communication of danger, your personality, past experiences, and prior knowledge all affect what you feel. Regardless of the actual damage in your body, you will only feel pain if your brain perceives a threat. You can have pain when nothing is "wrong," like the guy with terrible arthritis on his MRI but no history of back pain.

Since feeling pain is all about sensing danger, solving pain is all about restoring safety. How do we restore a sense of safety? Let's start with personality. Are you a high-stress or low-stress person? Type A or type B? Do you get excited by risky situations or do you prefer safety and stability? Our unique personalities, beliefs, and worldviews influence what we feel. Understanding the types of situations that make you feel safety or danger can help you identify where your pain comes from.

How about your past experiences? Sometimes our past experiences can sensitize us, and sometimes they can desensitize us. A small fender bender might be much more traumatic to someone who had recently been in a big car crash. That person would be sensitized by the experience. Let's say that the person in the fender bender was a professional stuntman. A little fender bender might not even elevate his heart rate! The stuntman had been in so many similar experiences that his brain was bored and desensitized to it. Drawing from a sense of safety in our past can translate even in new situations. If you know you have encountered danger in another area of your life and prevailed, remember that victory.

Nutrition and lifestyle choices also play a massive role in whether we are in a state of danger or safety. Poor food choices, poor sleep, strained interpersonal relationships, and job overwork can all contribute to a danger state. Conversely, take out the garbage and give your body an environment full of nutritious foods, rest, and healthy relationships, and it is only a matter of time before you feel like a different person. Why? If the body knows its healing system is preoccupied with other stressors, it knows it doesn't have resources available to deal with new problems. Thus, even tiny new problems are viewed by the body as big threats. Consider getting a $50 parking ticket if you had a $1,000,000 savings account versus if you were living paycheck to paycheck. The former is barely a slap on the wrist while the latter could be groceries for a week.

Knowledge is power. Simply knowing and understanding a phrase like, "Pain communicates DANGER; it does NOT communicate DAMAGE," can change how pain feels. Inside your brain, you have a medicine cabinet full of drugs more powerful than any pharmaceutical — without any side effects. Our brain can produce powerful opioids, pain-relieving chemicals, and lots of other feel-good stuff. The best way to access it is with knowledge of how pain works. So, finish reading this, and read it again. If you want to feel better, you're better off learning how to get the real stuff straight from the source — you!

Chapter 17: Don't Go It Alone

"You are the average of the five people you spend the most time with."

"Birds of a feather flock together."

"Guilty by association."

"Show me your friends and I'll show you your future."

"As iron sharpens iron, so one friend sharpens another."

"The godly give good advice to their friends; the wicked lead them astray."

There are so many quotes, idioms, and proverbs regarding our personal relationships that a complete list would be miles long. It's a fairly universal concept: We are highly influenced by those around us, and therefore must be careful about who is around us. Of course, this is easier said than done. You can't choose your family. Sometimes it seems like you can't be too picky with friends or coworkers either. So, what do you do when you want to get healthier but everyone you know is eating pizza?

The first step is often to look beyond your immediate circle of friends and family for inspiration. Just past these inner rings are new and exciting possibilities — groups of people who like doing things like eating kale and working out. More often than not, these are people just like you, with spouses and close friends who often prefer takeout to taking a walk. They've already begun to blaze a trail through the complicated jungle of balancing relationships and health decisions. Read blogs. Read books. Join a walking or jogging group in your community. It won't be long before you realize that there are lots of healthy people around you. You may be surprised by what you can see once the blinders are off!

The second is to be honest about who you keep around you so that you have an excuse to behave poorly. If you've got a friend with whom you tend to make your worst weekly health decisions, it might have more to do with you than them. Do you need that extra drink or serving of wings? Can you still keep up with your coworkers and get together for drinks without ordering the single worst thing on the menu? Be honest! Even if you get teased a little, no one worth keeping in your inner circle will ultimately criticize you for becoming healthier.

Third, be strategic about your time with family. If you've got a date night or vacation tradition that always indulges to excess, you need to change the nature of the date or vacation. There's nothing sexy about indigestion and nothing family-friendly about hangovers. If weekday dinners with your kids are always fast food, it might be time to remove a few extracurriculars and start cooking together.

Fourth, look for health allies. There are bound to be members of your family and friend group who are already healthy or who want to get healthier. They are probably looking for allies, too! Be intentional about spending more time with these wonderful people. It won't be long before you are drawing others into your positive group.

Finally, get professional accountability and guidance. Despite our best intentions, we rarely keep difficult promises that we make only to ourselves. When we determine that our health is a worthy investment, putting actual dollars into hiring a movement or nutrition coach can pay back exponentially. Additionally, having a true expert guiding you can make your efforts more productive and minimize the chance of stupid mistakes.

In other words: Don't go it alone!

Chapter 18: Build Strength For Longevity

If you're interested in longevity, you need to be interested in strength training.

But let's get one thing clear right away: When we say "strength training," we don't mean pumped-up muscles and endless grunting in a gym. Of course, strength training will give you a leaner physique and increased bone density. But it's so much more than that. We mean mastering your body's ability to control movement, generate power, and regulate other physiological systems. Let's break that down.

"Control Movement":

Movement is a skill that can be learned no matter what your body looks like. It is all about doing more with less. It is all about connection and coordination. Think Mr. Miyagi from the original Karate Kid. A bodybuilder with huge muscles may have good control when pushing a barbell above their chest, but that "strength" means nothing when life asks them to balance on one leg while trying to avoid a fall on black ice. Having big muscles can look nice, but they can also make movement sluggish and one-dimensional. Instead, coordinating hundreds of smaller muscles connected in adaptive patterns makes movement nimble and three-dimensional. It helps you handle life offensively and defensively. It helps you have fun with gravity as well as your grandkids. However, these chains can only operate if you have enough mobility to access them. If strength was a river, a stiff area in the body is like a dam: It dries up everything downstream. Thus, developing mobility goes hand-in-hand with developing coordination. Together you have masterful control of movement.

"Generate Power":

Once coordination and mobility are established, it is time to add power to the patterns. Power is a term used in the science of physics to define the rate of work done over time. Work is another physics term that defines the product of force and displacement. If you're not much of a physics buff, here's how that plays out in ways that you have personally experienced. Think about the difference between walking a mile and walking ten miles. Even if you are traveling at the same speed, ten miles took more "work" than walking one mile. If you can relate, you understand work. Now think about the difference between walking one mile and running one mile. The distance/displacement is the same. The work is the same. But the rate at which you accomplished the work was higher. The difference between what you experienced when walking a mile versus running a mile is power. If you can relate, you understand power.

Increasing your power involves increasing the work you can do while reducing the time it takes to do it. If you have ever said something like, "There just aren't enough hours in a day!" then learning how to increase your power may be just the thing you are missing.

"Regulate Other Physiological Systems":

Want better digestion? Strength train. Want better circulation? Strength train. Want a boost in mental clarity? Strength train. Want better sexual health? Strength train.

Most folks don't realize that strength training isn't just for your muscles and bones. It's for your whole body. Remember that the human body is more liquid than solid. Depending on where the liquid is and where it is being moved, a body can be at the pinnacle of health or the verge of death. Whether you are looking at the absorption of nutrients out of the small intestine and water in the large intestine, the circulation of cerebrospinal fluid in the brain, or the precise release of hormones and neurotransmitters, the movement of fluids in the body is arguably our most important physiological function. Think of a fast-flowing river versus a stagnant swamp. Moving water is a cleaner environment. The forceful contraction of muscles through full range of motion provides the displacement that helps to clear stagnant fluid, improve filtration, and introduce new materials throughout the body. These functions are just like the oil changes and fluid flushes in your car. Want to get your car to last 200k miles and beyond? Better change the oil regularly. Want to get to your hundredth birthday with aplomb? Better strength train!

So, why don't people strength train?

Could it be that the thought of strength training conjures up images of 1970s Arnold Schwarzenegger clad in spandex, sweaty, grunting, and comparing lifting weights to having sex? Or maybe it's the drudgery of doing the same machine circuit at Five Dollar Fitness while they play the same ten classic rock songs on repeat. To make matters worse, there are fallacies like "strength training is only for bodybuilders," "women who lift weights will get bulky," and "weight lifting makes you more likely to get injured."

There is so much information out there in the fitness world that we often don't know where to start. In a world of Instagram fitness celebs doing deranged exercises clad in very little clothing, it's tough to know what strength training really is. Add to that the bevy of different fitness approaches out there that all claim to be the right way and you've got a recipe for confusion. So, what to do?

First, know that doing something is nearly always better than nothing. Even though there are better ways to strength train, which we will discuss, going to the gym and doing the machines is certainly better than sitting at home watching Tiger King.

However, the fast track to making strength training a part of your life is to get a coach. Hire a reputable personal trainer or join a small group training studio (like ours), and have all the mystery removed. Even if your coach has an unnecessarily dogmatic approach, having

Chapter 18: Build Strength For Longevity

someone to cut through the noise and provide clarity on what to do is empowering.

Strength training can be anything from bodyweight exercises like pushups and squats, to weighted exercises like dumbbell chest press or kettlebell swings. You can also use resistance bands, suspension straps (like the TRX), or even things lying around the house like a milk jug or an unruly toddler.

Just get started. As you start strength training, you'll learn what works for you and what doesn't. You'll start to find which exercises are most important to helping you do the things you want in life. Continually tweak and make your strength training program better and build strength for longevity.

Chapter 19: Escape The Sedentary

Aliens have come to planet earth. Thankfully, these aliens are more like ET's parents and less like the ones from the scary Alien movie series. The government has assigned you as the head of a special task force designed to enlighten the aliens about modern-day American life.

As you begin to show the aliens around, they are flabbergasted. Earth's inhabitants live a perplexing existence. The humans live for short-term gratification. They seek comfort above all else, yet this very comfort is what ends up hitting them with a chronic disease making them VERY uncomfortable in the end. To find solace from the tiresome effects of gravity, the humans sit slouched in chairs all day long. Eventually their sitting leads to pain and discomfort for a body that is adapted to being stuck in a poor position. They use glowing screens to stimulate their eyes and minds to escape. They eat food that is easy instead of nourishing. Instead of climbing stairs or walking to get to a destination, they move about in warm little boxes (cars, planes, and elevators) being effortlessly whisked along.

The average American sits in their chair at breakfast, sits on the way to work, sits at work, sits on the ride home, and then sits at home and watches Netflix at night.

So, what's wrong with sitting? To quote Dr. Kelly Starrett, the author of Deskbound, "Recent studies show that too much sitting contributes to a host of diseases—from obesity and diabetes to cancer and depression—and literally shortens your life. The facts are in: your chair is your enemy, and it is murdering your body."[32] Sitting confines our body to a specific position for however long we are sitting. And the body "adapts." Muscles atrophy, the respiratory system learns to breathe in a compensatory sitting pattern, and the immune system weakens. Over time, with weakened muscles, poor breathing, and a shoddy immune system, our genetic code changes to express disease instead of health. This is why sitting is being called the new smoking.

The aliens are even more confused at the "exercising" humans. The ones running on a revolving mat or lifting things up and down repeatedly in a gym in the name of health. Our alien visitors would be befuddled at our conflicting behavior. Why would a creature that seeks comfort all day long punish itself with cardiovascular exercise and weight training?

---

[32] "Deskbound: Standing Up to a Sitting World (1): Kelly Starrett ...." https://www.amazon.com/Deskbound-Standing-Up-Sitting-World/dp/1628600586. Accessed 5 Nov. 2019.

Think of the person who heads out of their house before dawn to attend a 5 a.m. spin class, intense bootcamp, or to go for a jog. They punish themselves for 45 to 90 minutes, sweating their brains out in the name of health and longevity. Intense exercise (especially in a life of high stress) is a recipe for burnout, nervous system breakdown, and weight loss plateaus. Sitting nearly the entire day and then exercising at a moderately high pace for an hour or so is not how we've lived for thousands of years. Research shows that large amounts of sitting are not countered by a few hours a week of intense exercise.[33]

So, how are we meant to move?

Pre-agricultural humans slept until the sun came up, and moved all day. It was necessary for survival. It's been woven into our DNA. Without consistent and varied movement, chronic disease and the loss of independence and mobility are inevitable.

Instead, we need to entrench our lives with movement. We need to go for walks in the morning, stand at work, take breaks to walk during the day, and build movement routines into our lives.

After breathing, walking should be the most important movement in our lives.

Move often. Move well. Escape the sedentary.

---

[33] "Sitting time and all-cause mortality risk in 222 497 Australian ...." https://www.ncbi.nlm.nih.gov/pubmed/22450936. Accessed 8 Nov. 2019.

Chapter 20: Breathe Freely

Of all bodily functions, accessing oxygen is top dog. Go a few hours without a drink and your tongue will feel dry. Go a few days without food and your tummy will rumble. But go a few minutes without air and you will literally be on the brink of brain death. It's safe to say breathing is a top priority in the human body.

A threat to the respiratory system is Enemy No. 1, and will spur an immediate shift from parasympathetic (rest mode) to sympathetic (stress mode) activity. Due to our constant physiological dependence on respiration, the body will use the musculoskeletal system, the neurological system, digestive system — any system it needs — to make sure that the respiratory system is working. That's right: If your body is having trouble breathing, it will arrange your posture, your nerves, even the digestion of your Chipotle chicken bowl, in a way to facilitate breathing.

We need both the parasympathetic rest mode and the sympathetic fight-or-flight mode. Yet, due to overly stressful, sedentary lives inundated with toxic food and technology, people are stuck in sympathetic mode.

Our body's breathing strategy in sympathetic (danger) mode is different from its parasympathetic (safe) mode. In a safe, resting state, the body uses a muscle called the diaphragm to breathe. This muscle attaches to the front of your spine as well as the bottom inside part of your rib cage. With the low back and neck muscles relaxed, the rib cage sits in a position that allows the diaphragm muscle to dome. This is its happy place. Breathing in this position looks like gentle inhalation through the nose that causes all the ribs to expand and reciprocate from side to side.

This left-to-right rib cage reciprocation is complemented by our other reciprocating motions, such as walking. It is a beautifully designed, self-regulating system.

By contrast, when under stress, the diaphragm is pulled from its respiratory dome shape to become flat and taut to aid in stabilizing the spine as the body gets ready for fight or flight.

Without its primary respiratory muscle, the body must get oxygen somehow! Since the diaphragm can no longer work from below the rib cage to expand the lungs, the neck muscles take over from above, hoisting the rib cage up like a bird cage. Additionally, the muscles of the low back extend the lumbar spine to further lift the rib cage, allowing more lung expansion anteriorly (in front).

If this happens temporarily, there is no problem. Have you ever been swimming with a friend and had a competition to see who could stay underwater the longest? At first, holding your breath underwater had a surreal, almost peaceful quality to it. But as soon as the oxygen deprivation set in, your body immediately stopped digesting food and directed blood flow and neurological activity to the musculoskeletal system to propel you back to the surface. Once at the surface, you took a few gasping mouth breaths, hoisting your rib cage up, neck muscles bulging out. A few minutes later, oxygen levels had normalized and you were back to digesting and breathing diaphragmatically through your nose. No problem!

If this happens chronically, there is a big problem. We live in a world full of stressors, and each of them tells your body to go into danger mode. Whether by environmental pollutants, allergies and asthma, fear of failure, pressure to succeed in career and relationships, accidents, illnesses and injuries — our diaphragms keep getting taken out of a happy, domed shape and getting recruited as a soldier to defend against danger. Over time, our brains forget what a happy diaphragm even feels like! In a vicious cycle, our low back muscles get tighter and tighter, our upper back and neck muscles get tighter and tighter, and our ribs flare out in front. There is a reason people under stress say things like "I'm suffocating" and why a person finally at peace says they can "breathe a sigh of relief." Stress and breath are intimately connected.

Trying to calm down by "taking a deep breath" is ironic. The respiratory system under chronic stress is suffocating not because of too little air but too much! All those little gasping breaths IN add up, and it becomes increasingly difficult to get air OUT. This is why your ribs stick out in front (above your belly) — the lungs are hyperinflated, like balloons about to pop!

But wait — there's more!

It's not just low back and neck pain that result from stress-pattern breathing.

The dysfunctional overuse of low back and neck muscles, coupled with hyperinflated lungs and flared ribs, changes the position of the whole body, from your fingertips to your toes. Think of it this way: Your spine, ribs, and pelvis are the house that your shoulders, elbows, hands, hips, knees, ankles, and feet live in. If the house is falling over, it won't be long before the joints that live there fall over, too.

And that's not all! Remember earlier when we talked about the neurological and digestive systems? In a chronic sympathetic state, the neurological system is on high-alert, alarm mode.

Pain receptors become more sensitive than normal, and any injury is not only more painful but also more emotional and memorable. Meanwhile, the digestive system is all but forgotten. Its ability to break down food, absorb nutrients, and move waste out regularly and comfortably

Chapter 20: Breathe Freely

all diminish. At first, a person under stress will feel decreased appetite. Eventually, nutrient starvation will cause appetite to increase without regulation, spurring what is most often referred to as "emotional eating." Suffice it to say that dysfunctional breathing is a root cause of a myriad of health concerns that are often treated with costly surgeries, pills, infomercial supplements, etc. At this point, things may look a little bleak for us, but don't worry.

Let's get into the solution:

Respiration is the one vital function under both voluntary and involuntary control. This is a big deal. All of the sympathetic and parasympathetic responses we have been discussing are involuntary, or subconsciously controlled. In other words, you can't tell your digestive system to digest or not, nor can you tell your nerves how sensitive they should be. You can't put a finger on your pulse and through sheer willpower decide to change your heart rate from 72 beats per minute to 100.

But — and this is a big but — you can tell your respiratory system what to do.

Most of your breathing should be done through your nose. The nose is like your personal air filter. It cleans and warms the air before it goes into the lungs. It also has a relaxing, peaceful effect on the body and the nervous system. Breathe through your nose whenever possible.

Slow down. Change your breathing rate from 20 breaths per minute to 10 breaths per minute. This is key to the human design because it gives us access to our parasympathetic nervous system.

Focus on the exhale. Deliberately exhale through your mouth, getting all the air out of your lungs. Pause at the end of the exhale. Gently, and slowly, inhale through your nose. Repeat three more times and pay attention to how relaxed you feel after.

Match your breath with your movement. Forceful exertion, whether lifting a grandson off the floor or pushing dumbbells overhead, should be coupled with exhalation. The reason tennis players make those crazy sounds when hitting the ball is because a sharp exhale maximizes the power in their movement and protects their spine from rotational stress. Conversely, try to inhale when your body is relatively relaxed, for example, just before picking up your grandson. Trying to inhale when your body is under maximal tension will recruit muscles in your neck and back instead of your diaphragm.

You can breathe a sigh of relief. With a few minutes of intentional breathing each day, you can create lasting change in your pain, posture, and stress levels.

Chapter 21: Attain Alignment

"Do you think it's connected?" Marley asked curiously. Although she had come in for low back pain, Marley had just told me about some lingering knee pain, shoulder pain, and neck pain. "Oh! And sometimes my back hurts between the shoulder blades!" she added, scrunching her arm awkwardly to try to point behind her back.

Whether you have knee pain, shoulder pain, or neck pain — or all of them and more — there are a few root patterns that lurk behind nearly ALL of the different impairments we see. It's rare that multiple pain areas are unrelated (the exception would be if someone came in with low back pain, leg pain, and a rabid-looking Chihuahua latched onto their leg in a death grip. That person's back pain and leg pain would be unrelated, well, unless a second Chihuahua was hidden beneath their shirt...).

This is good news! It means you don't always need to see different specialists for every different thing wrong with you. Modern Western medicine was founded on the philosophy of reductionism, which basically seeks to solve problems by isolating them rather than connecting them. Reductionism was initially useful in developing vaccines for specific pathogens but later failed to successfully address modern ailments like chronic pain. When you understand how to change your alignment, you can often solve numerous problems at once.

How are most symptoms related? It all has to do with the asymmetries present in every human being. The two major sources of asymmetry in the human design are the internal organs and the hemispheres of the brain. Think about the last time you sang the national anthem or said the pledge. You put your right hand over your left chest because that is where your heart is! And it's not just the heart; most of our internal organs are asymmetrical, including the liver, lungs, stomach, and digestive tracts. These organs have different shapes, weights, and connections to the rest of the body. In the brain, the left hemisphere tends to be better at analytical and precision tasks, while the right hemisphere is better at creativity and artistic functions. Since the hemispheres control the motor function of the opposite half of the body, muscles on the right side of the body tend to be more controlled and dominant than the left (this is why most people are right-handed).

Before we say anything else, it is important to point out that this asymmetry is a good thing! It allows us a greater variety of skills and allows us to adapt to many different environments and activities. Much like a car needs to be able to turn right and left, our asymmetries allow us to navigate life's many roads. But what happens when we lose the ability to turn one direction? They say two wrongs don't make a right... but will three lefts?

Over the course of our life, we face many stressful, demanding situations. As children, we are more flexible in our approach to problem solving and will try many different methods of accomplishing the same task. The older we get, the more we tend to utilize only the path of least resistance. As crazy as it sounds, the way we pattern our movement on a day-to-day basis becomes so dominant that it is the functional equivalent of making three lefts to turn right! Not only is it inefficient, it causes uneven wear on our bodies in a predictable pattern.

Indeed, it is this very pattern that is behind nearly every impairment and pain problem that our clients face (besides the occasional rabid Chihuahua, of course). And it is correcting this pattern that leads to extraordinary outcomes compared to many traditional medical approaches. The solution is to restore a childlike flexibility in approaching different movement tasks; it is restoring the freedom to choose left and right, up and down, forward and back in any combination, at any time.

So, what is the pattern? And how do you correct it? The simplest explanation requires a basic concept of the rib cage and the pelvis. Think of them as two ovals stacked on top of each other. They should be able to rotate, side-bend, and tilt forward and backwards without losing orientation to a neutral center point. The "rib cage oval" positions itself primarily based upon breathing patterns and abdominal activation. The "pelvis oval" positions itself primarily based upon activation in the pelvic floor muscles and weight-bearing patterns (how the body centers weight over the feet). When breathing is stressed, anxious, or in any way chronically labored, the rib oval tends to tilt backwards, flaring in the front. Correcting its alignment has to do with stress management, diaphragmatic breathing, and activation of the side abdominal walls. Similarly, when digestion of food is chronically upset and when weight bearing occurs more towards the front of the foot and legs (or worse, when weight bearing occurs mostly on the tailbone due to excessive sitting), the pelvis tilts forward. Correcting its alignment has to do with improved nutrition and learning how to access muscles on the back of the legs and pelvis when standing and moving.

There is also a second, left-and-right dimension at play. This has to do with dominance of activity in the arms and legs, such as always writing with the right hand or always kicking a soccer ball with the left foot. It also has to do with the neurological and anatomical asymmetries. For example, the positional opposition of the heart on the left and the liver on the right predisposes the rib cage to greater flare on the left than the right. Finding and practicing left and right neutral requires a keen understanding of one's body and a lifelong practice of strengthening the less dominant patterns. In a perfect world, this would happen automatically and intuitively, but in our current, stress-filled, desk-bound world, it requires training and intention. However, these practices can be as simple as keeping the right shoulder elevated and retracted (farther back) when using a pencil or computer mouse rather than depressed and protracted (more forward). It can be as simple as standing more on the

Chapter 21: Attain Alignment

left foot than the right and keeping the left foot on the ground longer than the right when walking.

If any of you are Spiderman fans, you might remember Uncle Ben's famous line, "With great power comes great responsibility." Our asymmetries give us an incredible superpower: adaptation. Think of all the incredible and diverse activities humans are able to practice — from sewing to swing dancing, from cooking to climbing, from writing calligraphy to running marathons. But in order to do all of these things without over-using certain parts of our bodies and making them vulnerable to chronic injury, we must attain alignment.

Chapter 22: It's OK To Ask For Help

Why Is a Coach Essential for Getting Out of Pain?

We humans do not exist in isolation. Even the most capable, headstrong, and independent person still needs someone watching their back. Time and history prove again and again that plans succeed in the presence of wise counsel. Remember, back pain is just a symptom of a larger problem. The problem is that our typical lifestyles are incongruent with our body's design. Our lifestyles tend to develop around our personal paths of least resistance. If you want to move off the path of least resistance, there are going to be times when you need to be pushed, pulled, and even carried.

Whether your back pain had a definite start with a specific injury or came on gradually over time, your body needs a few key factors to maximize healing. One of those key factors is the growth and development of your entire movement system. Our bodies are designed to be challenged and built up not only when we are kids and teens, but all the way to the end of our lifespan. There is no age or stage of life where it is appropriate to stop growing in skill and strength. In general, one of the primary ways our bodies alert us to our behavior being out of line with our design is through pain. In other words, some of your back pain may simply be your body alerting you that it needs to be challenged again. This should be exciting, encouraging news.

While most of our patients come to us not even being able to dream of athletic feats like lifting heavy weights, jumping, or performing intense, cardiovascular exercise, by the time they have finished their initial course of physical therapy, they are looking at the future from a completely different vantage point.

In other words, getting expert guidance isn't only necessary for getting out of pain, but staying out of pain and pursuing the very best version of yourself.

Do You Want Our Help?

Our hope is for this book to be an amazing agent of positive change for your low back pain. Yet we know it's not realistic to fix every individual's back pain with what we wrote in this book. And that's OK. The book is meant to teach you why you hurt, to shed light on a better way to heal pain than pills, injections, or surgery, and to show you the principles you need in place in your life to be healthy and active. However, in order to pinpoint the best place for you to start, we need to know more about you!

You're unique. Your back pain problem is unique. And although implementing all the principles in the book and following the exercise program will do wonders for your health, it's tough to do on your own.

You need guidance, support, and encouragement on the journey.

So, if you're looking for help, we work with patients both in-person at our clinic in Glendora, California and online. Shoot us an email at back@villagefpt.com to learn more.

Conclusion

As both of us, Dr. Erik and Dr. Matt, sat together on the floor to decide upon a parting sentiment to leave the readers with, we came to the same conclusion: We've never read a book with a conclusion that we liked or that added anything relevant and actionable to the book.

So, instead of boring you with a summary of what we've already talked about or adding in another piece of information that we neglected to tell you earlier, we leave you instead with a smattering of rejected book titles. Feel free to write in to tell us which title you would have chosen.

Back Talk	Already taken. Sorry, Theresa.
Ditching The Boogeyman and Becoming A Boogie-Man	No explanation needed. It's just... terrible.
Back FAQ	We answered too many questions that no one in fact ever asked.
Back In Black	Royalty budget too small.
Back To The Future	Wanted to avoid almost dating mom.
Back To The Future II	Necessitates having already written the first book and titling it Back To The Future.
Back To The Future III	Necessitates having already written a second book called Back To The Future II that was written after a first book called Back To The Future, which was not written because of avoiding almost dating mom.
Bringing Sexy Back	Our ergonomic sex position guide was removed by the editor, and our wives.
Backed Up	Will make a better title when we write about GI distress.
The Backup Plan	Actually, this would make a pretty good title.
Broke Back Mountain	Not enough cowboy drama.
BackCountry	Original camouflage cover art didn't stand out from background.
Background	We really wanted this material to take the foreground.
I'll Be Back	The target audience for this book is humans, not cybernetic organisms from the future/Austria.

Appendix: Frequently Asked Questions

Despite our efforts to include all of the information you need to solve your back pain problem in a logical format, we know that some of you will still have specific questions. What follows are answers to those questions.

Do you have a different question that we did not cover? Feel free to reach us via email at back@villagefpt.com.

Who Can Help Me?

Finding help with low back pain is still a bit like the Wild Wild West. There are as many different types of practitioners out there who claim to help with back pain as there were cowboys in Billy the Kid's cowboy gang. It's tough to tell who is selling you snake oil and who genuinely has a method that will help you. I'll bet that you know someone who has had great success with massage, chiropractic, PT, and a surgery. I'd also be willing to bet that you know someone who has had a terrible experience with massage, chiropractic, PT, and a surgery. There are good PTs and bad PTs. The same is true for chiropractors as well as surgeons.

Here are a few tips to find a good practitioner:

1. Find an Expert

Luke Skywalker flew all the way to the Dagobah system to work with the famed master Yoda. And the result? He defeated the evil Emperor Palpatine, saved the galaxy, and restored balance to the force. Find an expert to work with, you also must.

You could look for someone who has written a book on the subject ;) or ask about whether the practitioner has helped people with your specific problem.

2. What's the Long-Term Plan?

Talk to the practitioner about how their skills are going to help you find long-term relief from low back pain. During the plan of care, they should not only be reducing pain but also helping you understand why the pain happened in the first place and what needs to happen to get you pain-free for good. In other words, all the adjustments and manual therapy in the world won't last unless you know what to do to keep your body in a good position.

In other words, does the program involve changing one's lifestyle so that the changes stick, or is it a quick fix?

3. Proof

You need some proof that the practitioner has been successful in the past with solving the same problem. They should have story after story of clients and patients just like you with your same complaints that they have helped. For stories of patients we have helped, re-visit the Introduction.

Should I Get a Massage?

"Massage therapy has been shown to have beneficial effects on varying conditions including prenatal depression, preterm infants, full-term infants, autism, skin conditions, pain syndromes including arthritis and fibromyalgia, hypertension, autoimmune conditions including asthma and multiple sclerosis, immune conditions including HIV and breast cancer and aging problems including Parkinson's and dementia."[34]

When you've had low back pain for a long time, there are observable changes in the brain.[35] The sensory (feeling) and motor (movement) cortexes become "smudged" and create a pain response with things that normally are not painful, like bending forward, walking uphill, or just standing still.

Massage provides a positive and different sensory experience that stimulates those same areas of the brain. As the brain is "plastic" and always changing, an influx of positive stimulus can create the kind of change in your brain that you need to break the cycle of pain.

However, alone, massage does not usually address the root cause of systemic dysfunction in humans. For more on the root causes and what to do, read the Principles section.

Should I Do Chiro?

Going to a chiropractor with low back pain is a mixed bag. The safest answer would be no, but we could say the same thing about the average physical therapy clinic — and we're physical therapists! We also know some really terrific chiropractors. What you want is someone who knows how to solve your problem from multiple angles and help you change your behavior so that you have a true, long-term solution and not just temporary pain relief. Be wary of chiropractors who rely heavily on passive modalities such as cold laser therapy and push expensive supplements. Look for someone who works with multiple health care disciplines and personally instructs high-quality movement. Look for someone who stands behind what they do, values your goals as much as you do, and acts as a teacher to help you master your

---

34   "Massage therapy research review - NCBI - NIH." 23 Apr. 2016, https://www.ncbi.nlm.nih.gov/pmc/articles/PMC5564319/. Accessed 4 Mar. 2020.
35   "Low Back Pain: The Potential Contribution of ... - NCBI." 2 Nov. 2018, https://www.ncbi.nlm.nih.gov/pmc/articles/PMC6900582/. Accessed 4 Mar. 2020.

body and be less dependent on them over time. Here's a rule of thumb: A good chiropractor should be able to solve your back pain problem without ever having to "crack" anything. They should be skilled enough to use manipulation as a tool in their toolbox rather than the proverbial solitary hammer.

Should I See a PT?

Sure! But shop around! Physical therapy is in a weird place these days. Back in the day, insurance companies made rather large payouts to physical therapists, and PTs responded by opening up clinics by the thousands. They didn't always do all that much, but they got paid for it. Eventually, insurance companies realized a lot of PTs didn't do that much, and started giving smaller and smaller reimbursements with greater and greater amounts of paperwork required to justify reimbursement. It was about this time that PTs started receiving a much higher level training (back in the day, a bachelor's degree sufficed, but now it is all the way at the doctorate level for minimum competency).

The result is that the average PT these days spends most of their time doing paperwork to justify their treatments to an insurance company that even under the best circumstances won't pay them enough money to allow the ideal treatment for their patients. In other words, physical therapists have had to find ways to bend the rules and exploit gray areas to get paid. This is why the average clinic will assign four patients an hour to a single therapist. That therapist must bill the insurance company of each patient for an entire hour (technically, it is 4 units, or a minimum of 53 minutes), even though they only spent a maximum of 15 minutes with the patient (and most of this time was distracted by relentless charting to stay on top of their paperwork for the day).

Perhaps this sounds like an editorial rant. The bottom line is that bureaucracy and greed have made it very difficult to find good physical therapy these days, even if you are working with a good therapist. You need not only a good therapist, but a clinic setting that focuses entirely on you. If you feel like the clinic doesn't take the best care of you, you're probably right.

Should I Go to My Primary Care?

Unless your main objective is to receive a prescription for one pill or another, there is very little reason to begin your search for back pain relief with your primary care physician. A physical therapist is trained to recognize any serious medical situations, related to your back pain or otherwise, and can refer you to a different care provider if necessary.

Conversely, one great reason to go to your primary care physician is to find out if there are any medications that you currently take that you could get off. One of the main reasons we send our patients to their doctors is to get off things like statins and blood pressure medication that make optimal health and performance nearly impossible. Most doctors see patients whose problems arise from an unhealthy lifestyle and, having no interest in living a healthy lifestyle, desire pills to mask their growing list of symptoms. If your doctor is adamant that you need to stay on something, seek out a second opinion. Look for physicians who break the mold and are passionate about patients who actually want to live healthy, vibrant lives.

How Can I Exercise If Everything Hurts?

This is a really important question! There is actually quite a bit of research that suggests continuing to exercise lightly is important especially when you are in pain. That said, if you can trace your pain to a specific motion, then you should generally avoid that motion for a time. In other words, if you are positive that your back pain started while stooping over to dig weeds, you're probably fine to walk, even if walking is uncomfortable. Just don't keep stooping over the garden. The one thing you absolutely do not want to do is hole up in bed for days or weeks. If you feel like you are totally immobilized, try to at least get onto all fours and slowly shift your weight backwards and forwards. If that is too tough, you can put your knees on the floor and your forearms onto a couch or chair and do the same.

Should I Do Mobility Exercises Like Foam Rolling and Stretching?

Definitely.

Here's a tip though: Don't make your objective with these types of activities to increase your mobility.

Wait, what? Do mobility exercises but not to increase mobility?!

Generally speaking, these exercises are great and often helpful for relieving pain symptoms. However, mobility is not straightforward. For example, many of our clients come in complaining that their hamstrings are tight and stiff. Many of them have been doing exercises to get more flexible, mobile, or looser hamstrings. However, when we actually assess them, it turns out their hamstrings are already way too long. The tightness they feel is actually coming from the position of their pelvis, which is pulling the muscle apart from its other attachments below the knee. Ironically, the cure for their tight hamstrings is actually to shorten and strengthen them, not increase their mobility!

Another important example of why mobility is not a straightforward concept is found at the spine itself. Often a segment that is stiff is immediately neighbored by a segment that is too mobile. Rather than the stiff segment, it is the mobile segment that gets extra wear and tear, causing irritation and pain, and eventually instigating an inflammatory response that makes the whole bodily region ache and feel... stiff!

The bottom line is that the body's need for mobility and stability can be tricky to understand.

On your own, it's better to make your objective to stimulate your muscles and joints and let your body's intelligence take care of what moves and what doesn't.

Let's put that into context and bring back the hamstring situation.

Do:

1. Foam Roll the hamstrings with moderate intensity.
2. Pair a mild hamstring stretch with a mild hamstring activation (e.g. gentle supine hamstring heel to ceiling, followed by heel dig or glute bridge).

Don't:

1. Use a foam roller or similar to beat your hamstrings into submission.*
2. Stretch your leg as far as it will go, hold it there as long as possible, and/or bob up and down like an old-school track athlete.

*We have a client whose catchphrase for any spot on her body that is bothering her is "I want to kill it." And she applies this desire liberally to her foam rolling if we don't gently persuade her to be kind to her body.

The reason the "Do" works is because it allows the body's soft tissues, joints, and related nerves and blood vessels to be stimulated without being threatened or permanently deformed. In turn, the body's innate healing system wakes up and starts to take care of the areas being stimulated.

The reason the "Don't" fails is partly because it puts you at risk for injury, but more importantly because it prevents your body's innate healing system from working properly. It would be like a five-year-old with a big idea of how to build a rocket ship out of cardboard and bubblegum walking up to a NASA engineer and saying, "No thanks, mister, I think I can handle this."

Should I Do High-Intensity Exercise?

The short answer: YES! (But with expert guidance.)

A lot of folks with low back pain have bodies that don't communicate well from joint to joint. Much like team sports, the human body has different players that need to be exceedingly good at their unique roles, but more importantly synergize with their teammates. Otherwise, "a chain is only as strong as its weakest link." Unfortunately, most therapeutic exercises either focus on only one joint at a time, or they are so gentle that the body never really gets ready for the rigors of the real world. Although these exercises play an important role in rehab, what we have seen clinically is the need for high-level, full-body exercises. We're talking barbell deadlifts, pull-ups, and all sorts of jumps and quick movements. This is not just true for young folks! Whether 18 or 80, there is no faster, more effective way to build a bulletproof back than learning how to push against ground and gravity.

Here's why:

When the physical tasks that you perform, including all your regular daily activities, only require sub-maximal effort, your body can get away with poor performance. It would be like (insert your favorite professional sports team) playing against (your high school team). The pro team could win without trying (unless it's football in Texas). Even if they were trying, their potential would still be diminished. Only in the presence of a worthy opponent is a team's true potential drawn out. It is exactly the same for your body. With only basic exercises, your muscles, joints, and nervous system have no reason to work together. When presented with a true challenge, powerful, coordinated movement is drawn out of you like water from a well. Our patients are often shocked at how strong they actually are when presented with a maximal lift. They are even more shocked when they begin to experience freedom from pain through these lifts.

Should I Do Cardio?

The short answer: yes! (But not too much.)

Healing is all about an efficient, effective inflammatory response. And that kind of inflammatory response is all about good circulation. There are few better ways to quickly boost your circulatory system than long rhythmic exercise — cardio! However, there are a few basic rules you need to remember to get those benefits.

First of all, you're trying to help your inflammatory system, not give it extra work. When you overdo cardio, you cause oxidative stress to your circulatory system that requires healing, and that means more inflammation. The easiest way to prevent this is to keep your heart rate in the aerobic zone. If you have seen those old-school fitness posters, this is sometimes called the "fat-burning zone." Basically, you want to keep your heart rate below 180 minus your age. This ensures maximum stimulation to circulation with minimum oxidative stress.

Second, you obviously want to avoid stuff that outright hurts. If your back hurts when you jog, don't force it! At the same time, try to avoid seated forms of cardio. Many back injuries can be traced to excessive sitting, so it doesn't make much sense to do more sitting. Try to choose the highest level exercise that you can do comfortably. Pool walking and/or water aerobics are great options if you are in severe pain. Walking on land with trekking poles is a great next level. Treadmills can be useful because you can control your use of handrails and incline to a sort of custom-fit walking experience. For a lot of folks, a slight incline can actually make walking quite a bit more comfortable than on flat ground. Ellipticals are also useful when walking doesn't work. However, their motion doesn't translate too well to the real world, so only use them if you cannot do any type of walking or if you just absolutely LOVE THE WAY THEY FEEL (shout out to my mom, who never stops talking about how much she loves being on her elliptical). I would hate to squash any activity that brings someone THAT much joy.

Third, don't look at cardio as the "end-all, be-all" of exercise. It's not the best way to lose weight, get strong, or increase stamina. It is a tool to help your body heal faster and get out of pain. A lot of our patients have been incredibly frustrated to have a pain flare up after getting too excited about walking, hiking, swimming, or fitness-machining. "I just wanted to burn some extra calories" are famous last words! Don't exercise to burn calories. Eat food to nourish your body and fuel movement that you enjoy.

How Will Breathing/Breathing Exercises Change Back Pain?

Oftentimes our patients balk when we begin breath work. Unfortunately, in our modern culture it is hard for folks to connect something as banal as breathing to profound healing. Yet breathing is the root of so much of what the body does, so it is hard to know where to start when divulging its merits. Let's try to break it down by body systems:

Nervous System:

We know that the nervous system is largely responsible for what we feel. Most of you are reading this book because you feel pain! Engaging the diaphragm helps to balance the sympathetic (stress) and parasympathetic (rest) nervous systems via stimulation of the vagus nerve. In turn, this helps decrease the sense of danger and fear that drives the pain experience.

Musculoskeletal System:

Most folks with low back pain come in and ask us how they can get a stronger "core." Even deeper and more central than our abdominal wall is our diaphragm. It is a sort of trampoline-shaped muscle that attaches to the lower part of our ribs and to our spine. It activates every time we breathe. That's over 20,000 times a day! You don't have to be a genius to figure out that something pulling on your lumbar spine 20,000 times a day can have a big effect over the years. Learning how to breathe correctly using your diaphragm is often the missing muscular key to solving low back pain for good.

Circulatory System:

Ultimately, it is your body's innate healing system that will take away your pain and injury. That healing system relies on circulation of blood to remove waste products and deliver new building materials. For many of these healing reactions to occur, oxygen must be present. When our breaths are shallow and only expand the top of our lungs, the oxygen transfer between the air and our bloodstream, called gas exchange, is inefficient. By learning how to breathe properly, air permeates our lung tissue all the way to the very bottom, where the richest networks of capillaries lay. Here, gas exchange is much more efficient, giving the healing system the oxygen it needs to do its miraculous work.

How Can I Make My Core Really Strong?

This is one of our most commonly asked questions. The truth about a really strong core is that the easiest way to get it is without doing any traditional "core exercises." No sit-ups. No crunches. No twists. In fact, many of these old-school core exercises actually damage discs. One of our patients had been doing 200 sit-ups a day for the last 30 years. We told him to stop, and by the next week, his back pain was already gone! Instead of these types of exercises that focus on moving the trunk, a strong core is built by resisting movement at the trunk while generating movement at the limbs. To put that in context, during a deadlift, the hips move while the spine stays still. For another example, during a standing chest press, the arms move while the trunk remains still. In order for this to happen, the body needs to be free to support itself. Locking yourself into an exercise machine that stabilizes your whole body prevents you from actively resisting movement in your trunk because the machine does it for you. Think of it this way, if your trunk would move if not for your active, intentional resistance during an exercise, you're doing some killer core work.

How Can I Fix Alignment in My Body? How Does Neutrality Affect Back Pain? How Can I Get My Body Neutral?

Another question we hear a lot around here has to do with bodily alignment. Most folks have a sense that if their body was lined up better, they would feel better. Conversely, they feel like parts of their body are crooked or twisted, and that is leading certain nerves, joints, and muscles to be pinched or pressed on. They notice that their left leg seems to behave differently than their right, or their right arm to their left. They may notice that one leg even seems longer or one shoulder is dropped lower. The good news is that the body is not designed to be perfectly symmetrical. In fact, the two hemispheres of our brains and the placement of our internal organs naturally bias us to certain asymmetrical patterns!

To start fixing alignment in the body, the first step is to understand how all the different pieces are connected in patterns, and then align not the body parts individually, but the patterns as a whole. When the body's patterns are all equally free and accessible, we call it a neutral state. Most back pain results from spending too much time in one pattern and not enough in the others. Getting neutral helps solve back pain because it allows the overused patterns to rest and gives the underused patterns a chance to get out and spread their wings.

About The Authors

Dr. Matt Klingler is a physical therapist and the owner of Village. He has a vision for Village to become a comprehensive solution for helping people optimize their health and live pain-free, vibrant lives. He and his wife, Nicole, have two amazing kids, Cooper and Chloe.

Dr. Erik Gullen is a creative genius. He does amazing things with his manual therapy skills, knowledge of the human body, and love for people. He is a doctor of physical therapy. He and his wife, Krissy, live in Glendora.

Health Advice Disclaimer

We make every effort to ensure that we accurately represent the injury advice and prognosis displayed throughout this guide. However, examples of injuries and their prognosis are based on typical representations of those injuries that we commonly see in our physical therapy clinics. The information given is not intended as representations of every individual's potential injury. As with any injury, each person's symptoms can vary widely, and each person's recovery from injury can also vary depending upon background, genetics, previous medical history, application of exercises, posture, motivation to follow their therapist, and various other physical factors. It is impossible to give a 100%-complete accurate diagnosis and prognosis without a thorough physical examination, and likewise the advice given for management of an injury cannot be deemed fully accurate in the absence of this examination from one of the licensed physical therapists at Village Fitness and Physical Therapy, Inc. We are able to offer you this service at a standard charge. Significant injury risk is possible if you do not follow due diligence and seek suitable professional advice about your injury. No guarantees of specific results are expressly made or implied in this report.

Made in the USA
Middletown, DE
21 June 2023

32469326R10125